Vertigo and the Vagus Nerve

Vagus Nerve Infection? Given the evidence of the involvement of infectious agents (virus or bacteria) in ME/ CFS, the prevailing view is that its symptoms reflect an ongoing immune response to infection, possibly because of immune system dysfunction. However, a recent hypothesis paper article goes much further; speculating that infection of the vagus nerve itself might be the cause of the illness.

Dr Van Elzakker from Tufts University in Massachusetts postulates that a viral or bacterial infection causes activation of glial cells (which support and protect nerve cells) somewhere along the vagus, which is a long, highly branched nerve travelling throughout the visceral organs, including the gastrointestinal lining, lungs, lymph nodes, spleen, liver and heart. Glial cell activation then produces inflammatory substances which bombard the sensory vagus nerve, sending signals to the brain to trigger a range of involuntary symptoms, including myalgia, fever, fatigue, sleep architecture changes and cognitive abnormalities. Importantly, when glial cell activation becomes pathological, as in neuropathic pain, the signals can become intensified and intractable, leading to chronic illness. According to the author; variation in ME/CFS between patients could be explained by the location of the infection along the vagus nerve pathway, the severity and duration of the body's response, and the type and severity of infection.

One advantage of this theory is that it simplifies the quest to find specific infectious causes for ME/CFS since any pathogenic infection of the vagus nerve can trigger the symptoms of the disease. But is the hypothesis true? Well, only experimentation can answer that question, and possible strategies include basic biomedical imaging of the vagus nerve pathway from the peripheral to central nervous system, or even functional neuroimaging studies if these are feasible.

BREAKTHOUGH
Journal of ME Research UK
Issue 18 , Autumn 2013, page 18

Vertigo and the Vagus Nerve
a medical mystery solved?

Merryn Fergusson, MCSP

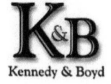

Kennedy & Boyd

Kennedy & Boyd
An imprint of Zeticula Ltd
Unit 13,
196 Rose Street,
Edinburgh,
EH2 4AT,
Scotland.
www.kennedyandboyd.co.uk

First published 2016
Text and Illustrations © Merryn Fergusson 2016

ISBN 978-1-84921-160-4

For my Mother
Diana Barthold

The Microbe

....But Scientists who ought to know
Assure us that they must be so....
Oh! Let us never never doubt
What nobody is sure about!

Hilaire Belloc

Acknowledgments

My grateful thanks to Lois Aitkenhead, Andy Platt, Angie Bythell and Gavin Aitkenhead for allowing me to write their labyrinthitis case histories.

Also to Letty for allowing me to write her case history of whip lash injury.

My thanks to Vari Drabble who read an early proof.

The work and teaching of Pete Emerson — Director of Rocky Mountain Manual Therapy Institute in Denver, Colorado — has been a major influence in my practise of physiotherapy.

Many thanks to Dr Twink Mellor for her help and advice regarding the tricky Autonomic.

For her tireless help in proof reading I would like to thank my ninety-year-old mother, Diana Barthold.

Finally, very many thanks to my fellow colleague and life-long friend Jane Bignell and to my fellow Spanish student friend Lois Aitkenhead for their time spent reading the first draft, and to Joy Pemberton-Pigott for her encouragement after reading the final draft.

Contents

Acknowledgements		*vii*
Illustrations		*x*
Introduction		*xi*

1	Neuron(e)	1
2	Lois	4
3	The Cranium	9
4	Cawthorne-Cooksey	14
5	Andy	17
6	Atlanto-axial	21
7	Angie	25
8	Gavin	31
9	Jane	35
10	Vagus	40
11	Twink	44
12	Vestibulocochlear	49
13	Ramsay Hunt	52
14	Abducent	54
15	Virus	56
16	Richard Hunt	59
17	Herpes Zoster	62
18	Epstein -Barr	64
19	Parasympathetic	67
20	Letty	70
21	Alpha Beta Gamma	73
22	Melvin Ramsay	78
23	Royal Free	82
24	Breakthrough	87
25	PACE Trial	92
26	Van Elzakker	95
27	Epilogue	99

References	*103*

Illustrations

...drawn to aid the reader's understanding.

Motor and sensory nervous systems	xii
Vestibular mechanism	3
The Cranium	8
Atlas and axis	21
Forward movement of the atlas	24
The underside of the cranium	33
The Vagus nerve	38
Vagus nerve	41
The medulla oblongata	44
Effect of malfunction of the dens	48
Mechanism of Ramsay Hunt Syndrome	51
Parasympathetic nerves	66
Mechanical malfunction of the dens	74
Van Elkazzer Hypothesis	89
Viral infection or mechanical malfunction	98

Introduction

Dizzy

Dizzy:- having a sensation of whirling and a tendency to fall. Unless you fall over, no-one can guess that you are dizzy.

It is a fact that medical professionals and patients have different ideas when they talk about being dizzy. Dizzy can mean vertigo, inner ear disturbance, labyrinthitis, light-headedness, loss of balance, orthostatic intolerance, feeling faint, and, feeling dizzy.

Mechanisms that cause dizziness can be circulatory, due to neck joint problems, or upsets of the inner ear. These in turn can be caused by trauma, infection, reactions to drugs, stress or a tumour.

Armed with the relevant information the doctor has to decide what sort of dizziness his patient is suffering from. However there are complications.

Dizziness can present with other problems; balance, migraines, nausea, fatigue, sweating, hearing loss, flickering eyes, tinnitus, and anxiety.

It also appears that some of the symptoms can actually be the causes; migraines can cause vertigo; fatigue can cause light-headedness.

I am a physiotherapist. I do not usually treat dizziness, vertigo and labyrinthitis, but when a patient recovered from labyrinthitis after one treatment, and this was followed quickly by three more cases, I was left with no option but to seek out the reason.

The journey led from Anatomy to Physiology, from herpes to research in Massachusetts into ME (Myalgic Encephalomyelitis). It led where I least expected, but it began with a case of patient who was dizzy.

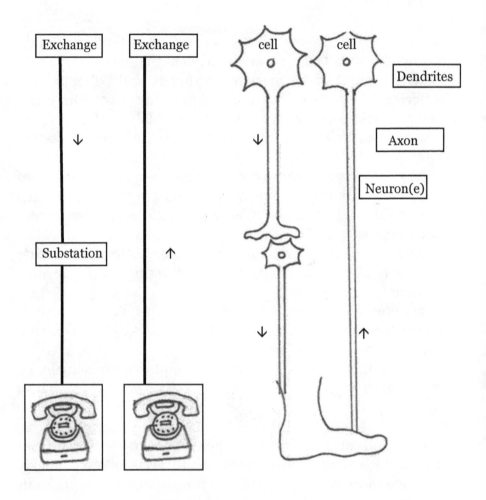

Exchange Exchange cell cell

Dendrites

↓ ↓ Axon

Neuron(e)

Substation ↑

↓ ↑

Motor and sensory nervous systems

Motor Nervous System sends outgoing messages
Sensory Nervous System sends incoming messages
Conduction of messages via nerves compared with a telephone
system, where the exchange represents the brain, and the
telephone represents a part of the body.

1 Neurone

This is a story which is held together by a nerve called the Vagus Nerve. Although the Vagus nerve is part of a system over which we have little or no control, it operates like any other nerve in the body. In Anatomy a nerve is called a neuron(e).

A Neurone is an electrically excitable cell that processes and transmits information. *In scientific sources the standard spelling is neuron.*

If a nerve to an organ is damaged it sends the same message to the brain as it would if the organ itself were damaged. I had to keep reminding myself of this fact when I surveyed the medical books and printed papers that were scattered over my dining table and wondered where to start with my most recent case.

A nerve is how the body transmits information. It consists of nerve endings or dendrites, a nerve fibre or axon, and a nerve cell or nucleus. Nerves conduct information to and from the brain. They are called motor if they send activating messages from the brain, and sensory if they send return messages to the brain. Motor nerves work like a landline telephone system. The telephone represents a part of the body. The nerve fibres are the telephone wires, and the telephone exchange is the brain. If a telephone does not work, it is not always because the machine is broken. The telephone might not work because the wires are damaged, or because the exchange is switched off.

An example of a motor nerve is the sciatic nerve. This long nerve extends from the lower back to the toes. One of its functions is to control the muscles of the ankle. There could be four scenarios for an ankle not to work. Firstly, if an ankle is sprained, then the foot will not move properly. This is similar to the problem of a telephone which is broken. Secondly when there is paralysis of the foot muscles or 'a dropped foot' caused by pressure on the sciatic nerve around the knee, such as could happen from a below-knee plaster, the axon or the telephone wire is damaged. Thirdly if muscles of the foot are weak due to injury in the lower spine because of a 'slipped disc' pressing on the nerve, the 'substation' of the telephone exchange is damaged. Finally if the foot is unable to move due to muscle spasm caused by damage to the brain so that it cannot send messages, then the telephone exchange is not working. In each case the foot does not work properly but the area of damage is different.

This sort of motor damage is easy to measure.

Sensory information is concerned with sensations that we feel, such as pain, heat, cold, and touch. Pain from a sprained ankle is registered by the brain via sensory nerves which come from the muscles and joints which are injured. However foot pain could be due to a 'slipped disc' in the lower back pressing on sensory nerves that have come from the foot but where the foot itself is uninjured. In each case the sensory information is registered by the brain as ankle pain.

It is always more difficult to assess sensory nerve damage.

When sensory information has been relayed to the brain and interpreted by the patient, a physician can only learn what it is like from the patient's description and cannot test it. The patient can only describe the strength of their pain, or the severity of their dizziness. The physician has no measurement for pain or dizziness

I have been a physiotherapist for many years, and I have regularly poured over Gray's *Anatomy* and other medical books which have accumulated, looking for details of muscles, joints and nerves. For these new cases of dizziness I had to extend my search to the internal organs of the body because they too have motor and sensory nerves. There are motor nerves from the brain telling the heart, lungs, gut, kidneys, blood vessels, glands and all the other organs that we are barely aware of, what to do. There are sensory nerves sending messages such as 'feeling queasy' or 'tired', or transmitting noise or light, touch or heat or cold, an awareness of our body in space, and especially in this story dizziness, to inform the brain about the state of our body.

Dizziness can be due to a number of reasons but the dizzy patient only knows that they feel dizzy. The information does not identify the trouble spot. Lois was the first of four dizzy patients diagnosed with labyrinthitis who came to seek my help in the autumn of 2014.

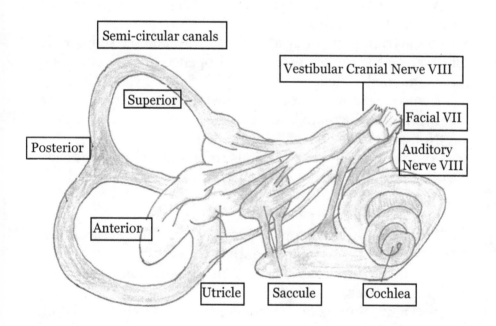

Semi-circular canals

Superior

Posterior

Anterior

Vestibular Cranial Nerve VIII

Facial VII

Auditory
Nerve VIII

Utricle

Saccule

Cochlea

Vestibular mechanism

2   Lois

In early September I met, as usual, with Lois for our weekly Spanish lesson. We had been studying together for about three years but our meetings had been less frequent since April. This was because Lois had been struck with labyrinthitis.

She described it as being inside a washing machine. She had spent many days lying in a darkened room with vertigo, nausea and brain fog.

Lois arrived punctually at half past two and parked her old blue car beside my old green one. I opened her driver's door. Lois remained seated.

"Como estas hoy?" I wondered how she was that day because her symptoms fluctuated.

"Not great to be honest." She replied.

"And your arm?" The previous week she had had difficulty writing. Lois held out her right arm and demonstrated her tremor.

"Not great." She repeated.

"When do you leave for the States?" Lois and her husband were due a post-retirement months' holiday.

"Seventeen days. I have no notion of going. I have not done any preparations."

I was naturally anxious on her behalf. With slight trepidation I said. "Shall we try a physiotherapy session?"

I am not sure what motivated her to say 'yes'.

At the end of the session, which took around an hour, Lois sat up and was silent.

Then she said, "My head is clear. My labyrinthitis has gone!"

We were both somewhat unnerved. At this point I had no explanation for what had happened and we were both aware that this recovery might be very temporary. We agreed to hold our collective breath and see what transpired over the next three days. We then proceeded with our Spanish lesson.

Three days later her head is still clear.

Lois insisted particularly that her head felt clear. All this was despite an episode of acute eye pain from a corneal ulcer which

4

had required attendance at her optician and at A&E. She said that she could not have managed the examinations prior to her physiotherapy session because she had to lie flat and tilt her head, and this would have exacerbated her symptoms.

Lois was mystified by the rapid change in her health. She had had labyrinthitis eight years previously and that episode had taken nearly a year to clear. To our second session of physiotherapy she brought the literature which she had been given in London. This included a detailed set of graded exercises, and two articles explaining the theory of exercises for labyrinthitis.

Labyrinthitis is an ailment of the inner ear, in which the balance mechanism which senses changes in a person's head position is damaged in one ear. It is possible to have bilateral vestibular deficits involving the labyrinths of both sides. They can be damaged by a virus, bacteria, a head injury, extreme stress, allergy or as a reaction to medication.

The ear consists of an outer and middle ear which are part of the hearing mechanism and an inner ear which houses the labyrinth system. The latter has three parts to it. Two are concerned with vestibular function or balance and one is concerned with hearing. The semi-circular canals, of which there are three, are set at right angles to each other and are filled with fluid. When the head rotates the fluid is left behind, but when the head stops it carries on moving. The movement of the fluid stimulates nerve endings which are interpreted by the brain as acceleration. These detect rotational movements. The central area has the utricle which detects upright posture and the saccule which detects sideways movements. The third part is the cochlear which is like a snail's shell and is concerned with hearing. Sound vibrations affect the fluid in the cochlear and these are converted into nerve impulses which are part of our hearing process. Injury to the labyrinth system causes balance disorders, vertigo, hearing loss and tinnitus (ringing in the ear). This was why Lois was given the diagnosis of labyrinthitis.

However, Lois did not only suffer from vertigo. There are quite a lot of other symptoms associated with labyrinthitis:

disorientation; nausea; light or heavy headedness; abnormalities of posture; instability and falls; neck pain; poor or blurred vision; poor head co-ordination; fatigue; low mood; agoraphobia (fear of the outside) and anxiety. Lois suffered from some of these but had been unaware that these symptoms were part of her condition. She eventually found out due to her own research.

In the worst cases people have difficulty in getting around, in cars, in crowds, on public transport and often need a walking aid and become housebound or wheelchair-bound. They are unable to go out alone and can only manage reduced domestic activities. They have difficulty working and have limited leisure activities plus a loss of confidence and difficulty in socialising. Lois was at times unable to go out and she dreaded car journeys because of their adverse effect on her symptoms.

Lois had been particularly distressed by her heightened sense of anxiety. This symptom lessened immediately after treatment. Her energy levels, which had dipped, and at times were very low, returned fully. She had even had symptoms of irritable bowel syndrome, and these too had cleared. She was able to travel in a car without experiencing 'sea legs' on arriving at her destination. She was able to ride her bike and do 'slaloms' if she wanted. After a fortnight she could drive, shop in crowds, and study and think straight, while only experiencing a little dizziness if picking raspberries. She could turn her head from side to side without dizziness and could stand still with her eyes shut. She found that she was back to worrying sensibly.

Lois had, I discovered when I assessed her, a very stiff neck especially when she tried to look upwards by dropping her head back. Her grip strength was reduced in both hands. She had a markedly clicking jaw on the right. She had restricted nerve movements in her upper arms which could be linked to restricted neck joints and cause her tremor. The reason that I attempted treatment was because these were the sort of problems that physiotherapy is designed to address.

There was, however, an unusual positioning of the joints just below her skull. When I held the mastoid processes behind her ears with my thumbs and placed the back of her head in the fingers of my hands, Lois's skull felt drawn and rotated backwards to the right to an extent that I had not felt in regular examinations.

My explanation was that the labyrinths were malaligned with each other triggering the vertigo. I thought that the two sides of Lois's skull and therefore the labyrinths were working asynchronously until I read up in detail about the semi-circular canals in Gray's *Anatomy*.

> The semi-circular canals are known as the anterior, the lateral and the posterior. The lateral canals of each side are on the same plane as each other, but the anterior canal of one ear is in a plane almost parallel to the posterior canal of the opposite ear. The planes of similarly orientated canals of the two sides showed marked departure from parallelism.

They were not placed synchronously anyway and the position of the labyrinths relative to each other was not the reason for Lois's dizziness.

I needed to find an alternative explanation because my next patient had no problems with the position of his labyrinths. Lois was in the States when Andy rang. Andy told me that he had had a bad back for years but that his main problem was labyrinthitis. Suddenly I had two cases in less than a month.

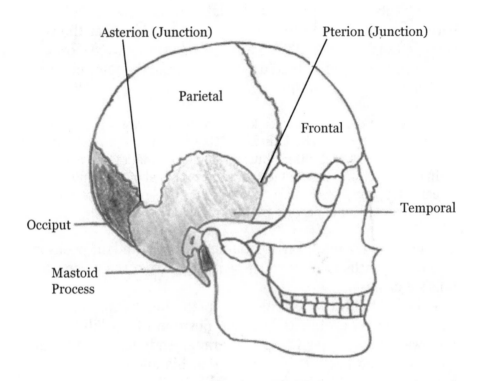

Asterion (Junction)

Pterion (Junction)

Parietal

Frontal

Occiput

Temporal

Mastoid
Process

The Cranium

3   The Cranium

The cranium is the anatomical name for the skull. In my first treatment session with Lois I began by mobilising the occiput, which is the rounded part at the back of the skull, with the upper vertebrae of the spine.

Then I had moved onto treating the sutures, the jagged joints that run all over the skull. Some felt too soft and others felt too resistant. Her joints felt especially resistant when I tried to 'lift' her forehead. On the other hand when I placed one hand under the back of her head and the other on a diagonal over her temple and pressed lightly from one hand to the other, her right side felt heavy. I was not aiming for any particular structure but just exploring and treating as I came across abnormalities.

During that treatment I identified several tight and tender neck joints and mobilised them using gentle oscillating movements. I was aiming to release any nerves that might be unable to stretch easily through her neck to her arm, so as to release the tremor. After that treatment the most noticeable change was in Lois's ability to drop her head back. This was a musculo-skeletal change.

It was significant that Lois had a strong reaction to her third treatment a week later when I concentrated on all the areas of her skull that Lois felt were tender or that appeared to me to be restricted. Following this she had twenty-four hours when her head hurt and her dizziness returned, although not the brain fog. This had been coupled with a late night but forty-eight hours later everything had settled.

The fact that her tremor had disappeared did tend to prove that her symptoms were not psychological, which is secretly what Lois feared. The treatment was very unlikely to have been a placebo. Lois herself commented later, 'There can be no possibility, in my view, that it was a placebo effect, as I was utterly convinced that my history proved that this condition was not structural, but in some way permanent, if not constant. I had not thought that physiotherapy might help.'

How does physiotherapy work? Fundamentally the therapist assesses which structures are not working, or not working correctly, and then plans a treatment. This is much the same as general medicine, except that physiotherapists use manual techniques instead of drugs or surgery. This is usually followed up by exercises to rehabilitate, or teach the body how to move normally again. On the whole the treatment is an active participation between the patient and the therapist.

Cranial work is essentially passive therapy. As a physiotherapist much of the information gleaned about a patient is by interpretation through our hands. When working abroad where there is a language barrier, treatment is, of necessity, predominantly passive. Whatever method is used the object is to increase movement; however, invariably, at the same time there is an increase in the patient's sense of well-being.

When I worked in Bosnia with victims of the siege of Sarajevo who were suffering, along with psychological trauma, physical trauma from those years of deprivation and maltreatment, it was easy enough to evaluate if their limbs or trunk needed attention. It was harder to assess how our physical treatments helped their psychological trauma, yet time and again we would, through the interpreter, hear how their anxiety had lessened, or their sleep improved.

The lessons learnt in Bosnia enabled me to expand my feel for the tissues, and sometimes just to follow where the structures led. Since Lois's condition was a new experience, I relied very much on what I could feel and treated her accordingly. If Bosnians had a reduction in anxiety with physiotherapy, there was no reason why Lois should not benefit as well.

It was not until two or three years before heading to Bosnia that I had considered the skull relevant to physiotherapy. As students we learnt in detail the anatomy of every part of the body, including the internal organs, their nerves and blood supply, but as far as the cranium was concerned we only studied the jaw, at the temporo-mandibular joint, and that because we could offer a form of deep heat.

An American, Pete Emerson, changed that. For a few years he introduced to the UK an innovative course of muscle energy techniques which covered all sections of the spine, and the final course covered the skull. Pete struggled to explain to officials at Customs why he had eight skulls, most of them reduced to their component parts, in his luggage. We had been set recommended pre-course reading which proved invaluable when he began by asking us, in pairs, to reassemble the skulls. Without some prior reading his references to zygomas and sphenoids might have overwhelmed us. In two days we had to absorb a whole set of new names and an even greater number of new techniques.

Before then I had not seen much call for cranial work. Physiotherapists in the musculo-skeletal field were rarely called upon to treat head injuries; these are the domain of those who specialise in neurology. After the course with Pete I did not have any idea to what depth or how often the cranial treatments should be administered, nor was it until two months later that I had a suitable patient to treat.

"Here's one for you." My colleague handed me a green referral card. "You can practise your new skills!"

The others in the practice had been mystified by my interest in this off-shoot, as they thought it, to our regular work. The case I was given was an elderly lady who had fallen twenty-two months earlier. Due to her age her reactions had been too slow for her to reach forward to break her fall, with the possibility of breaking her wrists, and she had fallen on her face resulting in two black eyes and a sore shoulder.

Subsequently she had been to her doctor complaining about her face. She had told him that she felt that "her tear ducts were blocked and that she could not do her work." Each time her doctor had replied, "But you have told me about that before." It was not until she told her story to a locum doctor that physiotherapy was suggested.

With my notes open on the floor beside me but out of sight of my patient, I gingerly attempted the first technique that we had been taught. This is an empirical movement with which all therapists in cranial work are familiar, the cradle vault. Carefully positioning the little fingers below the ears, and spreading the hands until the thumbs meet at an imaginary central parting at the parietal suture, the therapist has control of five of the bones that make up the cranium. With one under each fingertip, she or he presses gently with each in turn, like the keys of a piano, up and down the temporal, zygoma, sphenoid, frontal and parietal bones. In time the difference in the relationship between the bones is detectable, and moving rhythmically enables the therapist both to assess and to treat any area of resistance.

This was all that I had the courage to do on the patient's first visit as I did not know what the effect might be, and I spent the rest of the session mobilising her shoulder. At subsequent sessions I added in a different technique for her cranium, and her arm movement improved satisfactorily even if she had no other response. On her fifth session I added a technique that involved the nasal bones.

With two fingers of one hand the therapist hooks into the central arches of the orbits of the eyes, and then places two fingers of the opposite hand on the bridge of the nose. With an oscillating movement the nasal bones are distracted away from the orbits.

My elderly patient arrived, again with her husband of sixty years, for her sixth visit. She began speaking even before we had left the waiting room. "Sit down, dear. I need to tell you what happened. When I left here last time my nose started to run. It did not stop for thirty hours." She looked hard at me to make sure that I understood her. "And now" she said triumphantly, "I can do my work."

Later, when I scoured Gray's *Anatomy* to find out what I had done, I saw that, indeed, I could have cleared her nasal ducts. The sinuses drain through a small aperture at their apex, and the fall must have shifted the paper thin plates of the nasal bones just enough to close off the aperture used for drainage.

My patient was delighted with the outcome, and I was delighted that my time and investment in the course had proved worthwhile. Even so, I still thought of cranial work as specific for rare cases such as this one, until I went to Bosnia, where its use for treating the after effects of physical abuse, and for post-traumatic stress was critical. I began to discover that no treatment to the neck was complete if I did not include the cranium because it is so closely associated with the spine.

It is obvious that the spine and cranium and the sacrum are effectively one entity. No one part of the spine can be cured without all its component parts being treated as well, an approach that had been established by disciplines such as cranio-sacral therapy, but which I had taken a very long time to appreciate. I do not believe that Lois would have recovered as she did without the treatment to her cranium.

4 Cawthorne-Cooksey

When Lois had her first episode of vertigo she had conscientiously followed an exercise regime originally devised by Cawthorne and Cooksey in 1948. These were exercises which were graded from very small through to large general movements in twenty-five stages. The patient would do these exercises three times a day for five to ten minutes. The process could take a year. The exercises were designed to replicate the sensations of vertigo so that the brain could learn to re-programme itself. It was expected that the effects would be lessened if patients were exposed in a graded fashion to their symptoms, and to situations that they would normally avoid.

Lois had endured this programme, where she had to make herself feel worse for ten minutes three times a day, go in a car, be in a class with other people, and move in ways that made her vertigo worse, in order to get better.

In the early classes movement was only of the eyes following a finger up and down while keeping the head still. These progressed when the symptoms reduced to lying, rolling onto one side, sitting with legs over the side of the bed and lying on the opposite side, to whole body exercises with the eyes closed. Exercises were given as a class so that patients could support each other. Each patient kept a chart of his or her progress.

Cawthorne and Cooksey devised the labyrinth exercises in response to permanent damage to the balance mechanisms of the ear due to *trauma*. This would be either due to a head injury or surgery. They noticed that patients with vestibular disorders following head injury tended to become chronic; in other words their vertigo persisted and did not recover. The idea was to enable the brain to use compensating mechanisms to re-set their balance.

In the 1970s laboratory scientists surgically damaged the balance mechanisms of mice and then proved that they healed faster and that the brain adapted better if the mice were given visual cues and exercise. However in the 1980s these exercises were rolled out for all patients, even for *non-surgical* patients, with balance and vertigo problems and as eighty per cent improved 'it was assumed that the exercises had brought about the recovery'. A clinical trial compared the exercise regime with the effects of anti-vertigo drugs and the former showed greater improvement when the effects were evaluated 12-36 months later. There was no comparison with a control group, nor was any group offered musculo-skeletal physiotherapy, despite researchers noting that neck stiffness and pain often occurred with vestibular problems. It was thought that people did not move their joints because they were trying to decrease the unpleasant feelings of vertigo and therefore had pain.

Lois had been offered medication for her vertigo but later her London clinic advised her that these could exacerbate her symptoms. With the knowledge that Lois responded to physiotherapy it is not surprising that anti-vertigo drugs were ineffective. Nor is it surprising that exercises increased her symptoms because they were aggravating her neck which, in some way that I had yet to uncover, appeared to be causing her problems.

There is a pertinent footnote, in the light of what transpired later, to the Cawthorne-Cooksey regime and this relates to the psychological overtones that were associated with labyrinthitis.

Exercises were adapted and individual sessions arranged for those with severe symptoms, or those with a high probability of non-compliance, or for those who persisted inappropriately in believing that there was some sort of medication or surgery available to cure their symptoms.

It could be safe to say, considering the numbers suffering from the condition — the clinic in London has 50 referrals a month — that labyrinthitis is a common condition. Yet there is every reason to question the term labyrinthitis. Labyrinthitis means inflammation of the labyrinth mechanism; '-itis' means inflammation. Inflammation implies raised temperature around the infected area and often throughout the body, swelling of the area so that waste products can be removed and cells brought for healing, and finally a clearing up process. Patients with any of these symptoms would have received medication and would not appear in clinics for unexplained dizziness. There is no mention of illness, nor are the patients routinely prescribed medication for infection.

The theory behind the present Cawthorne-Cooksey regime is that the labyrinths have residual damage from an infection and this causes the lengthy course of the condition. There is no other condition of organs in the brain that has a similar pattern to this; neither middle ear infection, conjunctivitis, tonsillitis, meningitis nor the other brain infections. It makes the inflammation theory unlikely, especially in the light of Lois's rapid recovery.

In the absence of inflammation what might the problem be? It could be due to damage to the labyrinths themselves in the inner ear, or to the sensory nerve from the labyrinths, or in the nucleus of the nerve in the brain which is receiving information from the labyrinths.

> The dizzy patient is often treated by physiotherapists with good results. In some of these cases the symptoms are believed to be caused by obstruction of the vertebral artery in the neck. The dizziness and blackouts are thought to be due to compression of the vertebral artery as it winds through the canal that is formed between the facet of one joint and the adjacent facet of the joint below.

When considering the response that Lois had to manual treatment and the response of all those that have had successful manual treatment for dizziness, the Cawthorne-Cooksey regime and the premise behind it must be open to question.

It was to prove even more important to keep an open mind, however, when challenged with Andy's very different presentation of labyrinthitis.

5   Andy

Andy was an energetic forty-year old who ran his own kennels and worked with dogs. His labyrinthitis had begun in March but, unlike Lois, whose condition had come on slowly, Andy's had been sudden.

Andy said that on a Monday morning he had been feeling really good and had decided to clean his kitchen. He had done about three quarters of an hour's work when he felt that he was about to black out. He had time to ring for an ambulance before vomiting violently. The ambulance arrived within fifteen minutes and his symptoms continued while he was being driven to hospital. By the time he arrived he had lost the hearing in his left ear. All investigations that the hospital undertook proved negative, and Andy was sent home. For eight weeks he felt unwell. He was tired and slept for eight hours every night as well as having an hour's sleep in the afternoon. He had a severe headache, poor balance and dizziness. Alongside his deafness he had tinnitus, ringing, crackling, popping and an echo in his ear. His ear felt painful to touch and as if it was blocked with cotton wool. He had slowly recovered but in the last week some of his symptoms had returned.

Andy related that as a child he had had an operation for a cleft palate. When he was twenty he had had a serious car accident and fractured all the frontal bones of his skull. He had been in a coma for two days. Following this Andy had had two blood clots. He still suffered pain in his knees from where they had hit the dashboard. Andy suffered from backache all the time with some sciatica down his right leg. I later discovered that he had a nystagmus in his left eye.

Almost all of Andy's symptoms were common to labyrinthitis and this was his diagnosis.

People in our remote area of south-west Scotland are accustomed to travel quite considerable distances if necessary to work, go to market, to shop, catch a train, or to keep appointments. Andy had heard about me from a fellow dog handler. That is how it seems to happen. I will treat a teacher, and before long a trail of teachers find their way to my clinic. The same system works for foresters, builders, mothers with their children, friends and even members of an upholstery group.

Our house, a traditional farmhouse but without a farm, had been renovated and converted until only the end byre was left untouched. This we turned into an all-purpose room, but with its double doors leading directly onto the yard it was easily adapted into a treatment room. In acknowledgement of my advancing years I decided to reduce all pressure by allowing each patient one hour. This also tends to suit them since it reduces the frequency with which they need to attend.

There is a very steep hill leading up to the house and so I operate a simple system to help prevent my patients meeting on the narrow road. I allow the second patient to arrive and park before sending off the first. With new patients this is never a problem because they invariably arrive early. Andy was no exception.

During our first consultation I did a routine assessment. Andy had a multitude of minor restrictions throughout his spine, including reduced ability to look up and drop his head back, all of which made sense when considering his history, albeit that the accident had been twenty years earlier. He had restricted movements between some of the skull bones, especially around his ear, but he did not have the twisted presentation that I had found with Lois. His skull was not malaligned but I treated any relevant cranial suture and the joints of his neck immediately below his skull. When I gently stretched, or tractioned, his head and rotated it slightly, he felt pins and needles around his right eye which was the opposite side from all his other symptoms. I warned him that he might feel sleepy after his treatment, and as he lived an hour's drive away, to make sure that he stopped the car midway and walked around a bit.

When Andy returned for his second treatment he said that he had felt slightly better for two days, but was still dizzy and deaf. Generally he felt better because he had had no back pain, and his headaches had cleared up. On this occasion I again concentrated on his skull, working along the sutures and trying to free up the jammed joint where his skull met the upper joints of his neck.

On his third visit, Andy said that everything had been really good until two days previously when he had to get up suddenly in the night to attend to his little daughter.

He said that he felt 'wishy-washy'. All the ringing and crackling sounds had returned, and when he took his sweater off over his head he had nearly fallen over. He needed his eyes to keep his balance. His neck felt like cotton wool on the left hand side. Again he had a weird sensation behind his right eye.

Andy still felt wishy-washy after the treatment, and had suffered mixed symptoms, from severe ringing to a feeling of being bunged up. His sight was blurred in the mornings and distance sight was blurry all the time. He was, however, delighted that his headaches had gone, because they had been intense.

There is a form of vertigo that is known to respond to manual treatment. Andy had been onto the Internet and because he did feel easier if he dropped his head back and rolled it, we tried the Epley manoeuvre. This manoeuvre is used for Benign Paroxysmal Peripheral Vertigo (BPPV) where the episodes of severe vertigo are owing to the position of the head. BPPV is tested by doing the Hallpike test, where the head is turned to the right or left and then extended backwards to bring on the symptoms, and often a nystagmus confirms the diagnosis.

It is believed that particles or crystals in the posterior or anterior semi-circular canal are irritating the nerve endings and causing the vertigo. To resolve this, and to reposition the crystals, the Epley manoeuvre is performed. The person lies with their head turned fully to one side and with their head dropped as far back as possible over the end of a couch. After thirty seconds they turn to fully face the opposite direction. Then while lying on that side they sit up. In many cases the nystagmus and the dizziness disappear. This is different from the spontaneous nystagmus which occurs whatever the position of the head. Unfortunately the Epley technique did not make any difference to his vertigo and Andy's nystagmus also did not change throughout the treatments.

When he came for his fifth treatment Andy reported that he had probably had his best spell since March and although his deafness was unchanged his back felt 'brilliant'. He found that he could 'walk and text' at the same time. The ringing in his ears disappeared for a few days.

At this point his neck movements were all half range and the sliding movements of the nerves through his arms were still tight, especially on the right. The strength of both of his upper arms was reduced. His head where it joined his neck was tight on the right and his fifth neck joint needed attention. I treated all these areas and the upper part of his thorax, and as usual included his skull.

After this treatment Andy was generally better and as his condition had stabilised I was not sure that we could proceed further. He had no neck or back pain, his tinnitus and ringing were reduced and he no longer felt dizzy rising from picking something from the floor. He could now drop his head back three quarters of full range. He was happy with how he was feeling. His energy level was back to where it always used to be. His deafness and nystagmus persisted and his doctor was planning to send him for more investigations.

It was becoming reasonably clear that the labyrinths themselves were unlikely to be the cause of either Andy's or Lois's symptoms. Both Lois and Andy had responded to sessions of musculo-skeletal therapy which were unable to affect the labyrinths.

Andy was intrigued by anatomy, probably because of his interest in his dogs. He wanted to know more about the skull and neck joints, especially about the atlanto-axial joint, treatment to which had been pivotal to his partial recovery and to Lois's total recovery.

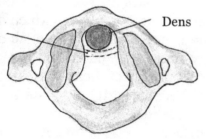

Transverse
ligament

Dens

ATLAS
First cervical
vertebra

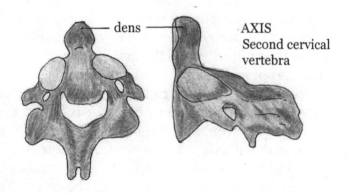

dens

AXIS
Second cervical
vertebra

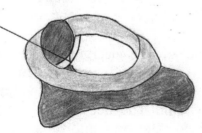

Transverse
ligament

Diagrammatic
position of
dens within atlas

6 Atlanto-axial

The cranium, the skull, is made up of many bones, of which fourteen are relatively easily accessible. It is like a football. The surface of the skull shows several jagged little sutures which is how the different bones adjoin each other. The central line, like a parting, is called the parietal suture; on either side, surrounding the ears, are the temporal bones which have small rounded projections, the mastoid processes, which can be felt behind the ears. These were the projections that felt so uneven when I examined Lois's skull. The forehead is the frontal bone, and the small dips on either side of the eyes are the wings of the sphenoid bone that passes behind the eyes and the nose and only comes to the surface at those points. Andy would have fractured some of these bones in his car crash. The occiput forms the back and the whole underside of the cranium and joins up with the sphenoid bone and the bones of the nose. In the centre of the occiput there is a large hole called the *foramen magnum* through which all the nerves from the brain converge to form the spinal cord.

The occiput sits on top of the atlas, the first cervical bone or vertebra, and the vertebra below it is called the axis. The axis is a ring of bone and it enables the head to rotate when the atlas and the axis act as a unit. All vertebrae — cervical, thoracic and lumbar — have solid bodies, except the atlas. An upward projection from the axis called the dens takes the place of a solid body for the atlas. There are strong ligaments holding these joints together, and of course, plenty of muscles to move them.

On the underside of the occiput, beside the foramen magnum, are two kidney shaped surfaces which neatly sit on two similar surfaces on the upper side of the atlas. This forms the occipito-atlanto joint. The head can drop forward into flexion, backwards into extension, and tip sideways as well as rotate. It was extension movements that were so restricted in both Lois and Andy's cases. Incidentally, there was the same loss of movement in two subsequent cases. The significance of this loss of movement becomes apparent when the mechanism is described in Gray's *Anatomy*.

When the head goes backwards, the occiput has to slide down the dens. The dens has a small waist so that the occiput can do this without putting pressure on the ligaments and adjacent structures. If the Occiput cannot tuck into the waist of the dens, then the head cannot go fully backwards.

To test whether a dens is intact the patient lies flat. With the fingers of both hands placed immediately under the skull where the occiput meets the atlas the vertebra is gently lifted upwards. If there is significant damage the patient will have neurological signs, might vomit, and have abnormal eye movements. This also tests the ligament that goes around the waist of the dens, called the transverse ligament. Fractures of the dens and damage to the ligament are associated with fractures of the facial bones. This made the test particularly relevant to Andy but it had proved to be clear and that a fracture of the dens or tearing of the ligaments holding it in place, was unlikely.

At every vertebral level nerves and blood vessels emerge to supply muscles and joints and the skin. If there was a transient loss of blood supply because the vessels were pinched by the adjacent joints, or because the vessels were constricted by spasm of muscles, this could explain dizziness or fainting. Reduced blood supply is the cause of some cases of dizziness.

Treating the atlanto-axial joint had cleared Lois's and Andy's dizziness. What could be the reason for many of their other symptoms clearing up as well? If the release of mechanical pressure caused by a jammed atlanto-axial joint cleared dizziness, it did not explain why Lois and Andy's other symptoms, such as tiredness, tremor, irritable bowel, sore joints and back pain, deafness and anxiety had also cleared up.

If Lois and Andy's dizziness was not caused by constricted blood supply, and was relieved by removing pressure at the atlanto-axial joint, it suggests that their labyrinthitis was not due to problems in the inner ear in the labyrinth mechanism. This means that the 'telephone' was working. If that was the case then it left the axon, the telephone wire, or the nerve nucleus, the exchange, as the trouble spots.

A coffee meet-up with a friend, Angie, at around this time, coincidentally opened up a new window on labyrinthitis.

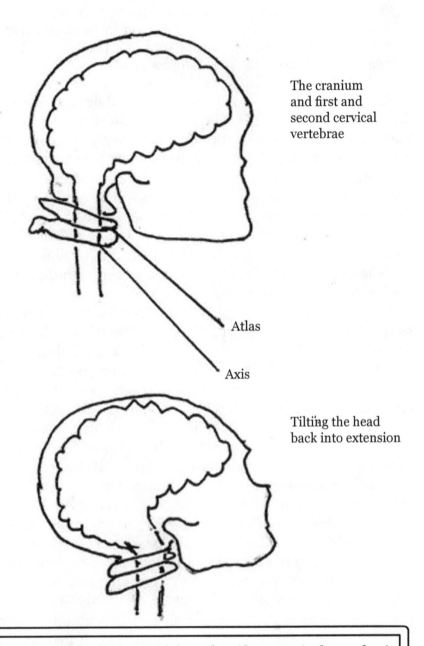

The cranium
and first and
second cervical
vertebrae

Atlas

Axis

Tilting the head
back into extension

Forward movement of the atlas (first cervical vertebra)
and axis (second cervical vertebra) as the cranium moves
to tilt the head back.

7   Angie

A few days after Lois had flown to the States, I met up with Angie. Angie and I had trained together, and then, twelve years after qualifying, had discovered that we lived within fifty miles of each other. Angie had recently retired from working and so I did not often bother her with 'shop'. However, because Lois's reaction to treatment was so dramatic I could not resist talking about it. Angie, therefore, had to sit and listen to the whole saga, including assessment and treatments, because she was a physiotherapist, and only a fellow therapist would have the patience.

She remembered the Cawthorne-Cooksey exercises which we had learned about in our training, but she expressed her doubt about their efficacy. She had good reason. Angie reminded me that about twenty five years previously she had had her own experience of vertigo. One morning she had been unable to get out of bed, and even clutching onto furniture could not make her way unaided to the bathroom. Consultant appointments had queried Multiple Sclerosis but all tests, including an MRI on her brain, had proved negative. She said it had been like a very bad sea sickness that had lasted about a year.

Angie then divulged that recently she had experienced uncomfortable symptoms which she reflected were similar, but not nearly so pronounced, as those of her first assault. She admitted that she had been particularly tired and stressed due to family problems. Would I have a look at her?

Angie said that she felt 'wobbly' regarding balance, as if she did not 'trust her feet'. Her anxiety levels were at around five out of ten but that it was more as if she was being irrational. She felt her brain was fogged at a level of six out of ten. She said that her energy levels could be as low as two out of ten. Sometimes she had no option but to sit down for half an hour and after that she would be able to continue. She felt queasy at times, her jaw clicked and jammed, and she had intermittent strange sensations in her face. She had a tendency to lose her voice. She hated going to the dentist because of the position of the headrest and how her jaw behaved. She had had some occipital headaches recently and she was not usually a headache sufferer.

Out of curiosity we decided to meet later that week in my treatment room.

Angie had restricted neck movements especially side bending, which she had lost completely, and extension where she barely had half of full range. She had weakened muscles in her shoulder and her hands on both sides, indicating some neck joint involvement. She had movement restrictions at the atlas and axis and at the sixth and seventh joints. The plasticity of the some of the nerves in her arms was lost. When I looked at her cranium, she had a tender occiput. Her temporal bones on both sides had tender areas as did the posterior section of her parietal suture. When I felt the diagonal movement, her head felt heavy. The heaviness had been behind Lois's right ear. With Angie, it was the left.

During that session I treated all her cranial joints by moving them gently one on the other. This resulted in an increase in her neck side bending, rotation and extension. The plasticity in the nerves of both sides improved. I then addressed her atlas, axis, and the lower cervical joints and her neck extension almost gained full range. The strength of her shoulder muscles on both sides improved although her grip strength was unchanged. We must have taken about an hour and when we had finished Angie said that she felt taller and lighter.

A week later Angie reported that, apart from a 'hiccup' due to a family problem when she was very tired, she had had a very good spell.

On our second meeting a fortnight later Angie had wrenched her fifth and sixth ribs trying to lift a suitcase onto an overhead rack in the train. Before I treated her I reassessed from the last session.

Angie said that her balance was nine out of ten, and her energy ten out of ten. Her brain fog was nine out of ten except for one episode. She still had a small loss of extension of her neck but her side flexion was full range on the left and slightly restricted on the right. Her nerve mobility was slightly reduced on the left probably due to the rib injury. Her cranium was well aligned with a slight restriction on the right occipito-atlanto joint. I treated her cranium, occipito-atlanto-axial joint, her upper cervical and her affected ribs, and added some nerve mobilisations.

Two weeks later she said that she was completely fine unless she was particularly tired from commuting to see her invalid relative. Could Angie's symptoms have been due to stress and anxiety as the literature often suggests?

How can a physician or a therapist decide if a symptom is the result of a physical abnormality or the result of psychological stress?

Some years ago a patient came to my clinic with recurrent incapacitating elbow pain. After some time the decision was to operate to relieve pressure on a branch of the radial nerve. It may or may not be significant that due to poor communication her dressing was not removed for inspection for over a week. Six weeks after the operation the patient had gained no relief from her pain. She went on to develop a condition resembling reflex sympathetic dystrophy where pain and swelling persist due to irritation of the nervous system that is not under voluntary control. I received a direct phone call from her Consultant, an almost unheard of occurrence, enquiring, not about our rehabilitation regime, but about the woman's personality. The inference was that she was malingering with some view to compensation. With the knowledge that she was a conscientious manager of a local television rental shop where part of her job was to lift and carry televisions, who valued her job highly enough to pay for private treatment, I was able to refute the idea that my patient had a psychiatric overlay. Reflex sympathetic dystrophy is a known complication of operations especially of the arm, and there was no need to look further. Nor, in fact, could the Consultant have prevented its development as there is so far no known cause for this condition, but it was curious that he wanted to 'blame' the patient for not recovering.

The level of anxiety experienced by the majority of our patients could be described as 'normal'. Life is rarely plain sailing but our bodies and minds are equipped, usually through time, to cope. The physical body builds up immunity and our mental health builds resilience through experience.

There can be very few people attending an out-patient clinic who could be said to have been stressed enough to cause a permanent pathological anxiety state, when compared with what was meted out and endured by Bosnians in Sarajevo. In my experience there in that summer of 2004, where people were exposed to real trauma over a prolonged period of time, the question of anxiety as a cause for a physical illness, what is called psychosomatic, did not seem to arise. Our clients recovered their health, both mental and physical, from treatments that were purely physical. We had no language in which to communicate and there was no psychotherapy available.

Prior to that work, my colleague and I attended an induction day which was held in a Women's Rape Refuge in the centre of Edinburgh. The leader of the organisation explained that the siege of Sarajevo lasted just under four years and was the longest siege in modern warfare. They warned us about unexploded mines, the continued political unrest, the financial straits of the government and the strong fundamentalist Muslim presence from abroad.

The Bosnians that we were to meet were, of all patient groups, the most likely to suffer from post traumatic stress disorder and associated psychological symptoms.

The overall experience of working with patients in Sarajevo reflected its architecture in that they were a charming but their past had left deeps scars. The clients had been under siege and isolated, at the mercy of physical abuse, torture, rape, starvation, cold and constant fear. Every one of our patients had suffered; the woman with no relatives left alive, women and young girls isolated in high rise flats surrounded by areas of destruction at the mercy of the Serbians. This was unremitting mental and physical torture. We did not encounter malingering or pain due to anxiety and they would have good reason for these labels. These labels as causes can be used in our surgeries for unexplained syndromes such as labyrinthitis, chronic fatigue, and non-specific back pain. Psychosomatic pain and malaise were not labels used in Bosnia, where they might be expected to be found.

Our traumatised Bosnians accepted sleeplessness, nightmares and traumatic stress as part of the fallout from the war, but fortunately many responded to manual therapy regardless of technique. Therapists took massage, Indian head massage, Bowen technique and other alternative therapies to Sarajevo, and into this mix we added joint mobilisation and where possible, rehabilitation exercises. To no one technique could their recovery be attributed, since no therapist stayed longer than two weeks, but over a six month course offered every year, the clinic delivered exciting results where not only did their pain diminish but clients began to be able to sleep.

The secretary of the Federation of concentration camp victims was one who had been helped. He came to the clinic to invite the therapists to his house for a day to relax at the weekend. He sat down in the office and to begin with spoke in German to one of the therapists before switching to English. He came originally from Mostar, a town renowned for being separated into two religious groups, one on either side of the bridge, who had lived peaceably for many years. The war destroyed the bridge and a greater part of the Muslim sector. He had not gone back. He had been with five others in a darkened room for eight months. As he spoke he crossed his wrists as if to indicate that they had been tied. His mother lived in Srebrenica, where one of the worst massacres had taken place, and had been missing since the war, as had nine family members. All the while as he was talking he was working his hands. The tragedy of the situation was that the six of them who were captive knew their gaolers.

If stress caused psychological illness or psychosomatic illness then we would have expected a high proportion of stress-related psychological or psychosomatic disorders in Sarajevo. The effects of labyrinthitis on the lives of patients are extremely unpleasant; however the effects are unlikely to cause mental health illness. There should be, therefore, only a relatively small proportion of labyrinthitis patients suffering from stress-related factors, yet the literature suggested that most cases had psychological factors. These factors were consistently present and are therefore significant. Was the anxiety found in labyrinthitis, in fact, psychological or did it have a physiological basis?

Even although Gavin, the fourth labyrinthitis patient, was in a more than usually stressful situation, it hardly compared in severity with the circumstances of any one of our Bosnian clients.

8　Gavin

The common factor in the treatment of Lois, Andy and Angie was the range of extension at the atlanto-axial joint. If altering that cleared up dizziness and vertigo it was unlikely that there was anything amiss with the labyrinth mechanism itself. The telephone was working. This left the wires and the exchange.

In all three cases the response to treating a mechanical problem had been a reduction in symptoms of dizziness, energy levels, brain fog, and anxiety. Was it possible that these were caused by some musculo-skeletal dysfunction rather than the other way around? Was it possible that movement of their necks really was causing their vertigo?

At this point Gavin with a different presentation of labyrinthitis or dizziness arrived in my clinic and his case helped, later, towards understanding the significance of the occipito-atlanto-Axial region. This pointer was not towards the telephone wires or axons, the nerve fibres that wound their way through the brain and spinal cord, but to the exchange and the cell nuclei themselves.

Gavin requested an appointment to see if anything could be done about his increasingly distressing face and neck symptoms. Starting originally around his mouth and chin, Gavin was experiencing pins and needles which were now spreading to his nose and all around his eyes. He said that it was there all the time and that it was exhausting. To trigger the symptoms he would sniff, and wrinkle his nose which felt blocked.

His eyes felt as if they were always screwed up and as if he was frowning constantly. He said that his eyes looked different and were almost bloodshot. He felt that he wanted to keep them closed and that 'his eyesight seemed not to be right'. He had become sensitive to bright light, but he could not wear dark glasses because the frames irritated his skin.

His mouth was numb and swollen as if he had been to the dentist. If he rubbed his hands over his face then the sensation stopped temporarily. Recently he had odd cold-sore-like blisters on his lower lips which had not developed into cold sores. He had a metallic taste in his mouth and his salivary glands felt overactive, yet he had a dry mouth. He was queasy but did not know if it was hunger or whether he would be better not eating.

When Gavin chewed, his ears felt blocked. His hearing was diminished and if he rubbed his right mastoid process he was aware of water inside his right ear, meanwhile his left ear hummed. In the last two months his brain was fogged or fuzzy and he was worried about concentration because he had stopped at a green light.

Gavin's energy levels had been at six or seven out of ten for the last six months. His balance was eight out of ten and he suffered from dizziness on rising to stand which increased his facial symptoms, as did sudden movements like brushing, when on the ice, Curling. Gavin said that his skin was clammy and worse after eating. He was not 'a headache person' but he was on the edge of a headache all the time.

Getting to sleep was a problem which it used not to be. He disliked bends in the road when driving because he had spells of vertigo.

Gavin had been diagnosed with leukaemia, but without the need for treatment. He said that he lost patience more easily and that his anxiety levels had increased. He admitted that the diagnosis might make him anxious.

The Consultant had said there was no indication that these symptoms were due to his leukaemia.

Gavin was sixty-two years old and very fit as his job was maintenance at a small school where physical activities were emphasised. He was not overweight and ate healthily. The only trauma of note had been five years previously when he had been clearing some undergrowth and a large branch had struck him on the nose. He had been thrown to the ground and had passed out momentarily. His face had been a 'real mess'.

The main findings on examination were limited neck movements especially extension and side bending, various dysfunctions at his cranial joints, and some in his cervical vertebrae. The initial consultation had been lengthy and there was only time to treat his cranium. This resulted in a slight increase in range when he tilted his head backwards.

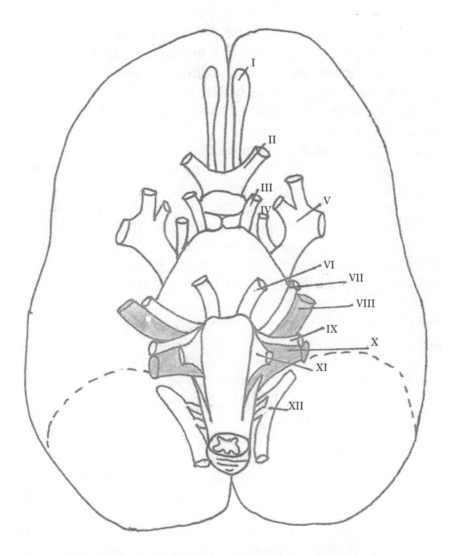

I	Olfactory	II	Optic
III	Oculomotor	IV	Trochlear
V	Trigeminal	VI	Abducent
VII	Facial	VIII	Vestibulocochlear
IX	Glossopharyngeal	X	Vagus
XI	Hypoglossal	XII	Accessory

View of the underside of the Cranium showing the twelve pairs of cranial nerves.

At his next session Gavin said that the pins and needles were less but that everything else was unchanged. However, after this session there was a marked improvement and the pins and needles had again reduced. He said that he 'felt better in himself'. Over the next sessions he continued to improve unless he was very tired.

Gavin's case was more complicated than the other three. The sensations that he was describing appeared to be due to a mix of nerves, but what was causing these nerves to play up was not clear. Sensations such as tingling in the face and odd feelings in the eye and nose, all pointed to irritation of the cranial nerves. These are nerves that are specific to the functions of our senses — hearing, seeing, smelling and tasting — and include actions and sensations of the face and throat, as well as controlling balance.

There are twelve cranial nerves which, as their name suggests, start in the brain and not in the spinal cord. They have their cell nuclei, or power houses, in the brain. To see them properly you have to turn the skull upside down and then look at the underside of the brain. The cranial nerves are numbered from the front.

The cranial nerves which could have caused some of Gavin's symptoms were the third cranial nerve, the oculomotor which controls some of the movements of the eye; the fifth cranial nerve which is the trigeminal, one branch of which, the maxillary, sends messages of sensation like pins and needles from the face; the seventh is the facial which controls the muscles of the face and taste and glands in the nose, mouth and throat; the eighth is the vestibulocochlear which controls hearing and balance; and the ninth, the glossopharyngeal which controls the throat, salivary glands and taste buds.

This list covered many of Gavin's symptoms but, apart from the fact that all these nerves were quite close together on the underside of the brain, at this point it was impossible to understand how so many cranial nerves could be affected. Yet there was no other explanation for these most unusual sensations.

9　Jane

This would not have been a story without Jane. Jane and I met at Occupational Therapy College but we both left and, in different parts of the country, went to study Physiotherapy. It was Jane who, knowing that I was free to travel again after three years of looking after my teenage son, suggested that we try our hands at working abroad. Her offspring no longer needed her and the idea of voluntary work overseas had always attracted us.

Jane has three scars in close proximity; one from an appendicitis which became infected, one from a caesarean, and one from an elective removal of her ovaries. It was this last operation that began the havoc. From the day after her operation Jane has been at the mercy of a system that will go into overdrive, sending her heart rate from a sedate sixty beats a minute to two hundred, causing palpitations, sweating, and feeling just awful, a state that she can be left in for more than a day. I was once the unwitting perpetrator. Any stretch on the scar tissue in her lower abdomen would set off these symptoms, and while practising some manual technique I pulled her right leg, albeit gently, but that was enough. She said that, coincidentally, she had had a windsurfing accident which had affected the base of her skull and upper neck vertebrae.

Jane's area of expertise for a long time was cardiac rehabilitation, she then worked for fifteen years in the same field as myself, that of musculo-skeletal manual therapy, until she moved into oncology. Our regular telephone calls invariably include a discussion about any current physiotherapy case that we are struggling to untangle.

"What news?" she asked.

This was an occasion where she might have regretted such a question because before long I was in full flow.

"Slow down" she begged as I rattled on about the four recent cases of labyrinthitis. "Tell me about the link with the neck."

"The movement loss in each case was most noticeable when the head extended, and recovery reflected improvement in head extension." I told Jane, and went on to explain. "When the occiput moves down the dens, it seems that it is important that it can slide into the waist of the dens. Since the foramen magnum is a circle of bone, if the occiput cannot tuck in while moving downwards it compresses the structures inside the foramen. In fact the whole occipito-atlanto-axial joint including the transverse and alar ligaments are probably involved."

"Yes." Jane sensed that there was more because this was not a particularly remarkable phenomenon, physiotherapists have successfully treated dizziness using techniques to mobilise that area. "Where are you going from here?"

"All four patients were suffering additional symptoms which the literature on labyrinthitis labels as psychological factors: these are fatigue or tiredness that is unusual, anxiety, low mood, and agoraphobia."

"What are you thinking?"

"If these psychological symptoms disappeared with their physical symptoms the theory behind the Cawthorne-Cooksey exercises needs to be revisited. What could be causing the vertigo *and* all the other symptoms? If the labyrinthitis had been due to a viral or bacterial infection it is strange that none of these patients have been offered antibiotics and none have mentioned a fever."

"As you said, Lois and Angie had slow onset, and this suggests that it was unlikely to be an infection. Infections rarely have a slow onset. Had any of them had a head injury?" Jane asked.

"Andy had, years ago, and I suppose Gavin had to some extent. None of them had been offered treatment for residual musculo-skeletal problems, and in the Cawthorne-Cooksey trial, although they had noted that some people could not do the exercises due to painful joints, none were treated."

"Stress is difficult to evaluate, but tension in neck muscles by affecting the joints could, as it possibly did in Gavin's case, set off symptoms." Jane pointed out reasonably. "But only a mechanical fault could resolve labyrinthitis with the speed that Lois's cleared. It is unlikely that all four of these people had anxiety and other visceral symptoms prior to their labyrinthitis."

"What symptoms would you expect from damage, infection or irritation of the labyrinths themselves?" I asked.

"The same as if they were irritated on a merry-go-round or on board ship, loss of balance and sickness. Andy did not even complain of nausea, did he, after his initial attack? There has to be another explanation, and ideally, it would cover all the symptoms that they all experienced." Jane then suggested. "It could be some problem affecting the autonomic nervous system."

This other nervous system works in tandem with our voluntary nervous system and operates automatically. In order to cope with every day functions automatic mechanisms are needed. These control the fluid matrix of the body and keep it hydrated, oxygenate the blood via the lungs, and enable digestion and absorption of food for energy. The Autonomic system has to ensure that the body is supplied with the correct blood flow at the correct blood pressure by regulating the heart, that waste is excreted, body temperature maintained, reproductive behaviour controlled, and defensive mechanisms against viruses and bacteria mobilised.

In the background this system has to make sure that the body can recover. It does this by controlling the circadian rhythm, the daily routine of the body, which allows sleep for growth and repair of cells.

The sympathetic nervous system is the emergency system of the autonomic nervous system. It comes into play whenever we encounter situations that arouse 'fear, flight or fight'. If we are about to be chased by a lion, to quote Sapolsky in 'Why Zebra's Don't Get Ulcers' we don't wait around to digest our meal. We are aware of the effects on our bodies when preparing for a race and the concept of an adrenalin rush. In these situations the sympathetic system, firing on adrenalin, alerts the organs that will enable us to respond. Adrenalin is poured into the body and these organs, the heart, lungs, limbs and brain are stimulated appropriately.

Voluntary Nervous System   Autonomic Nervous System

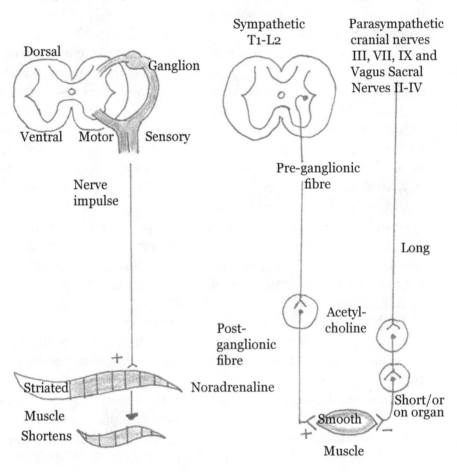

Smooth muscle:-
If + excitatory exceeds -
then smooth muscle shortens.
If - inhibitory activity exceeds +
then smooth muscle relaxes

Sympathetic:-
Can be increased by
a hormone from
the adrenal medulla

Parasympathetic:-
No system can increase
its activity. Does not
necessarily all work
at the same time

> The Vagus nerve (Cranial X) is the major part of the parasympathetic branch of the autonomic nervous system.

The parasympathetic nervous system is less studied than the sympathetic nervous system. It is responsible for 'rest and digest' or 'feed and breed'. Instead of being activated by a hormone in the blood, it is activated by acetylcholine which is transmitted from nerve to nerve.

"So what about these other symptoms?" I countered.

This is where Jane, before she too set off for USA, said enigmatically, "Look at the Vagus."

On her voyage of discovery as to the cause of her own symptoms, Jane had researched the possible effects of irritation of the Vagus nerve. What Jane was sending me to look at was the effect of disruption to the parasympathetic nervous system which is more or less totally under the control of the Vagus nerve.

10 Vagus

"Lois has been telling me about the Vagus nerve." Gavin said to me during one treatment session.

"Yes" I answered expectantly.

"She tells me that it is in my head." Gavin continued.

"Yes." I said.

"That it is in the top of my head."

"Oh dear! I have not done a very good job at explaining." As Lois is Gavin's sister I knew that the message would be passed back. "The power house of the Vagus nerve, the nucleus, is in the head, but the nerve goes just about everywhere inside the body except the limbs. It is called the wanderer."

"What exactly does the Vagus nerve do?"

The Vagus, the tenth cranial nerve, is noticeable by its size. It is the largest and most extensive of cranial nerves. From the brain it sends branches up to the ear and to the covering of the brain in the occiput and joins the facial and the glossopharyngeal. The motor component of the Vagus goes to the heart where it slows down the rate. It constricts the airways of the lungs. It controls the movement of the stomach and enables secretions for digestion but it also closes off the sphincters. It does the same throughout the gut and it controls as far as the first third of the large intestine. The Vagus also controls the blood vessels of the abdomen, as well as the liver, pancreas and glands above the kidneys. The sensory component of the Vagus informs the brain of the state of the viscera.

Unlike the sympathetic the parasympathetic does not work altogether all of the time. The Vagus is a major player in the parasympathetic system. When a nerve impulse reaches its destination it releases the chemical transmitter acetylcholine. The acetylcholine release may bring about contraction or it may bring about relaxation of these involuntary muscles. As soon as it is produced acetylcholine is removed by cholinesterase.

Could the symptoms, other than balance and hearing, suffered by Lois and the other patients be due to the parasympathetic action of the Vagus nerve?

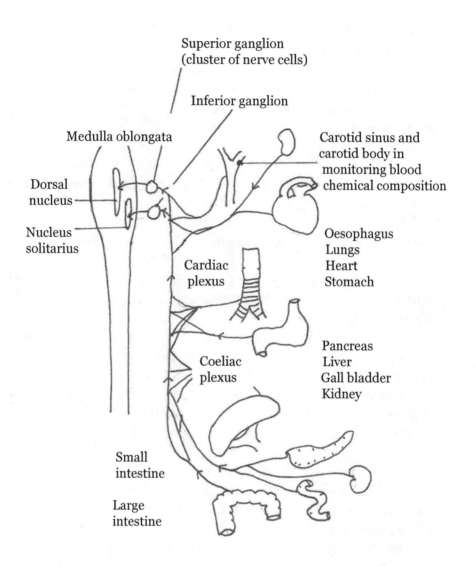

Superior ganglion
(cluster of nerve cells)

Inferior ganglion

Medulla oblongata

Carotid sinus and
carotid body in
monitoring blood
chemical composition

Dorsal
nucleus

Nucleus
solitarius

Oesophagus
Lungs
Heart
Stomach

Cardiac
plexus

Pancreas
Liver
Gall bladder
Kidney

Coeliac
plexus

Small
intestine

Large
intestine

Vagus nerve

Most of the information sent from the viscera (internal organs) to the brain is from the Vagus nerve.

Fibres terminate in the dorsal nucleus and tractus solitarius in the medulla oblongata.

The Vagus could cause headaches, due to its meningeal branch in the posterior occipital fossa. It has no influence on the eyes, and therefore could not cause Andy's nystagmus. The branch from the Vagus has only a small input to the skin of the outer ear, and does not affect hearing or balance. It could cause Angie's 'lost voice' if the pharyngeal and laryngeal nerve were affected.

The effect on the carotid body is uptake of oxygen by the blood. The Vagus has a slowing effect on the heart so that response to exercise requires more effort.

The effect on the lungs is constriction of the airways and a poor response to oxygenating of the blood which would affect exercise.

If gastric juices were increased then the person could feel nauseous. There would be more secretions from the bile duct, also causing nausea.

More secretions from the pancreas means that sugar absorption would increase and the person would be low in sugar and therefore low in energy. Lois wondered if this was the cause of her constant desire to eat, which she said was different from comfort eating, and which left her when her labyrinthitis cleared up. Gavin, too, said that he did not know if he was hungry or if he were better not eating.

In the digestive tract from the oesophagus to the large colon, the parasympathetic increases the digestive juices which leads to a fast passage of food through the intestines, and poor absorption of foodstuffs.

The effect on the coeliac plexus is to increase gastric juices so that the gut is flooded, however it also constricts the sphincters which allow passage of food from one part of the gut to the next, and a kind of irritable bowel is set up.

If there is increased activity of the large intestine then there is an increase in water absorption and the person tends to be constipated.

But, there was a snag. There is a right and a left Vagus nerve. Once they exit from the back of the skull, they only meet when they are in the thorax. If one side was compressed or irritated as it began its journey down the vertebrae, even if it was caught just as it emerged at the occipito-atlanto-axial joint, the other Vagus is capable of maintaining the status quo. There would be no effect from one side being interrupted.

Only if there was a mechanism which affected both Vagus nerves would Jane's suggestion, that the symptoms were due to parasympathetic activity, hold up.

What might cause the parasympathetic to play up?

As Jane was still in the States, I decided to contact Twink.

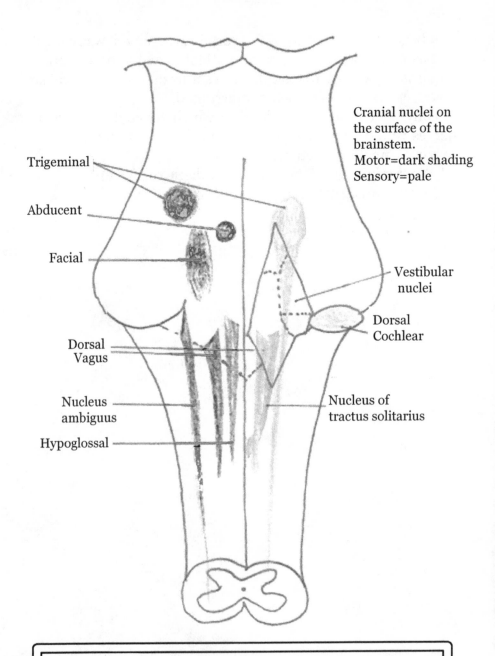

Cranial nuclei on the surface of the brainstem.
Motor=dark shading
Sensory=pale

Trigeminal

Abducent

Facial

Vestibular nuclei

Dorsal Cochlear

Dorsal Vagus

Nucleus ambiguus

Hypoglossal

Nucleus of tractus solitarius

The medulla oblongata showing close proximity of Cranial Nerves VI, VII, VIII and X.

Dorsal Vagus, Nucleus Ambiguus and Nucleus Tractus Solitarius are all nuclei of Vagus Nerve (Cranial X).

11   Twink

"Twink!"   I emailed. "I have a case of Labyrinthitis that responded to treatment of the upper neck. Looking at the anatomy it seems possible that the Vagus is in some way involved. I am hazy as to the relationship of the sympathetic to the parasympathetic and the role of the Vagus nerve." Twink was a doctor who had specialised in psychiatry and whose husband was a researcher into nerve physiology. Despite fielding the needs of two tiny children, Twink responded promptly.

"It is a little while since I was a student."

However, she had been a student a great deal more recently than I had. "The two systems work synchronously with each other, one switching on as the other switches off."

Homoeostasis is the name for when the body is in balance and it is aiming for homoeostasis all the time, hence the see-saw action of the autonomic system.

Twink went on, "If the parasympathetic was down-regulated then the sympathetic would be up-regulated. It is probable that the treatment Lois received to the upper neck area had up-regulated the carotid sinus, which would up-regulate the Vagus." This would be irritation to the axons or the telephone wires of the Vagus.

However, it was Twink's comment about up-regulating the parasympathetic that resonated.

If the Vagus was up-regulated, then it would be overdoing things. If the sympathetic overdoes things then the body organs work even harder and the body '*races*'. If the parasympathetic is overdoing it then the body organs would be *slowing down* excessively. How would the body respond to this? How could the body control a system that is sending the body into freefall? It could only be by activating the sympathetic which would start things up again to try and regain normality. This would be why Jane was flushed, sweating, her heart racing and her pulse going crazy. Why she twice ended up in hospital with palpitations and yet had nothing the matter with her heart. Jane's body appeared to go into sympathetic overdrive, but was in reality responding to a drop in Vagal activity, in an effort to return to normality or homeostasis.

What might be the effect of a body that is slowing down towards danger point? Anxiety and panic, possibly. A dangerously slow heart rate, breathing that slows down to critical levels, a digestive system that rejects food, blood pooling into the central viscera to keep the vital organs alive leaving the exterior, the face and limbs, pale. If the brain is short of blood and oxygen then thinking becomes clouded. In Gray's *Anatomy*, under applied anatomy, it describes what happens when the radicular nuclei of the Vagus are damaged.

> The functions of the Vagus may be interfered with by damage to its radicular course in the medulla or during its path through the cranium. The symptoms produced by a non-functioning of the nerve are palpitation, with increased frequency of the pulse, constant vomiting, slowing of respiration, and a sensation of suffocating.

Close to death, and frightening, but here we had a scenario where both the Vagus nerve axons and the nuclei were implicated and that was in the medulla.

This described, in part, what Andy experienced when he had to call the ambulance. It could explain the loss of energy, the anxiety, and the brain fog that Lois and the others complained of.

Where were the nuclei, the power houses of the Vagus? Obviously they had to be in the brain tissue because the Vagus is a cranial nerve. As we see above, Gray's *Anatomy* locates them in the medulla in the brain stem where the brain begins to gather into a stalk and eventually becomes the spinal cord.

The Vagus has four nuclei. The most significant of the nuclei, the dorsal nucleus lies in the central grey matter of the medulla oblongata. The four nuclei are on the surface of the medulla at the posterior or rear surface. The nuclei of the right and left Dorsal are close together in the centre with the hypoglossal nuclei on the inside and the nucleus ambiguous on the outside. Incidentally, a fact that became important later, the nuclei of the Vagus are at the same level as the nuclei of the trigeminal and the vestibulocochlear. The nuclei vary in length but they all extend for some considerable way (the medulla is three centimetres long) up and down the medulla.

The position of the nuclei of the Vagus was also significant. The medulla oblongata, at the level where the dorsal nucleus of the Vagus is located, is at the level of the atlas. It is on a transverse plane that corresponds to the upper border of the atlas and the middle of the dens. This area of the medulla is considered closed because it is within the spinal canal, and therefore pressure in this area from any injury would be greater than further up the medulla or other areas of the brainstem. The nuclei of the Vagus were exactly where the pressure seemed to be exerted when Lois and the others were trying to tip their heads back into extension.

Co-incidentally, it was the same movement that is performed by the Epley manoeuvre that has such success with BPPV.

But it could not be coincidence. At the atlanto-axial joint the Vagus nuclei are beside each other, so pressure on one would, more than likely, cause pressure on the other. At this point both Vagus nuclei could be simultaneously irritated and this would cause the parasympathetic nerves to be affected throughout the body.

At last there was an anatomical area where the nuclei of the Vagus were in close proximity and where both could be affected by an injury together, and the area was at the atlanto-axial joint where treatment had been directed in all four cases of labyrinthitis. Any pressure within the medulla at that level would have an impact on the nuclei that are sitting on the surface. These would then be compressed against the posterior ring of the atlas. Any limitation of the ligaments around the dens, preventing the brainstem from sliding comfortably beneath the dens when the head extended, would compress all the tissues of the brainstem in that vicinity.

Twink had not only explained how the parasympathetic would slow everything down, since its function was to maintain homeostasis and settle the effects of an excitable sympathetic, but she had pointed the way to the anatomical position of the nuclei of the Vagus and a possible explanation for the Vagus to malfunction.

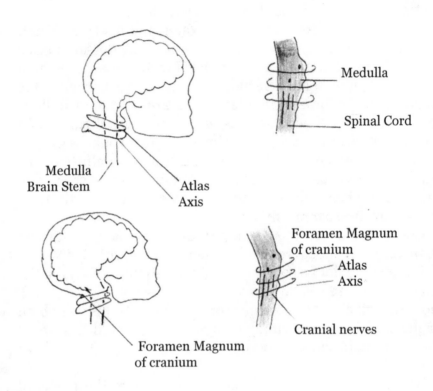

Medulla

Spinal Cord

Medulla
Brain Stem

Atlas
Axis

Foramen Magnum
of cranium

Atlas

Axis

Cranial nerves

Foramen Magnum
of cranium

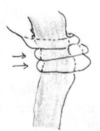

Pressure on medulla oblongata
by atlas and axis

Effect of malfunction of the dens.

12   Vestibulocochlear

Finding that the Vagus nuclei were located in the medulla did not tell the whole story. It accounted for some of the labyrinth symptoms but did not explain Andy's deafness, tinnitus and nystagmus, or Gavin's pins and needles, or the balance and vertigo in all the cases. The proximity of the vestibulocochlear nuclei to the Vagus nuclei, and the possibility that any injury that affected the Vagus could also affect the vestibulocochlear led to the next stage.

What did the vestibulocochlear do?

The eighth cranial nerve is concerned with balance and hearing. Balance mechanisms in the semi-circular canals and the utricle and saccule connect via the vestibular portion of the nerve. The snail-like hearing mechanism connects via the cochlear portion. Both send messages to the nuclei in the medulla in the brainstem at the level of the dens of the axis. From the medulla messages then connect with eyes, neck, limbs and the cortex of the brain to keep the body's equilibrium. From the medulla messages are directed to the relevant portion of the brain to interpret sounds as hearing.

However, the vestibular portion of the vestibulocochlear nerve, if damaged, could, without the labyrinths themselves being in any way involved, cause vertigo. In the same way as a person can feel pain in their foot due to nerve damage elsewhere when the foot itself is unaffected, so it could be possible for a person to experience vertigo without the balance mechanism itself being affected. It explains why, if caused by mechanical pressure, once the area is treated and the compression is lifted, the system returns to normal. The person regains their balance. The nerves are, in fact, only temporarily out of action.

The vague or possibly Vagus symptoms, and those of balance or possibly vestibulo symptoms, predominated in the cases of Lois, Angie and Gavin. The involvement of these two nerves did not explain the symptoms of nystagmus and the complete loss of hearing in his left ear which were unique to Andy.

However, a disease process, the Ramsay Hunt syndrome,

is a syndrome that involves both deafness and vertigo and is, curiously, a distinct syndrome of both the vestibular and the cochlear portions of the eighth cranial nerve.

"The Ramsay Hunt syndrome might shed some light on Andy's plight." I suggested to Jane during one of our telephone calls.

"Why are you so bothered?" Jane asked. "We have helped loads of patients get better over the years, some faster than others. Why are you so obsessed with these cases, especially Lois's case?"

"When Lois was developing her tremor I was very worried. Her vertigo was distressing and we did not think that there was any help available for that. However, when she recovered instantaneously, instead of feeling pleased, I felt really angry."

"Why angry?"

"Because Lois had had to put up with so much misery, she actually said that life was hardly worth living. Because so many people have gone through exercise treatment that involved replicating symptoms of vertigo. Because they had to do the exercises for so many months with little guarantee of recovery. I feel obliged to do something."

"It is not anyone's fault. The research said that it was the correct treatment."

"But we know now that they only saw what they wanted to see. They ignored the musculo-skeletal signs. They limited their research to comparing just two aspects, the exercises and drugs. They ignored what the patients were telling them."

"There are probably other conditions out there where we are doing the same thing." Jane rationalised.

"This is a chance to make a difference."

"A research paper?"

"We are in no position to write a research paper. We've no back-up, no papers to give an evidence base, and there are years of studies proving the opposite. The only way is to tell their stories."

"And start by finding about Ramsay Hunt syndrome?"

"Exactly!"

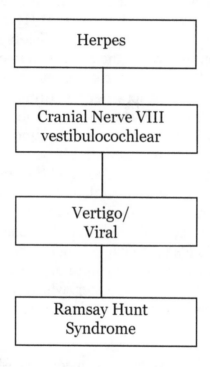

Mechanism of Ramsay Hunt Syndrome.

Herpes attacks vestibulocochlear nerve causing vertigo and viral symptoms.

13   Ramsay Hunt

Ramsay Hunt was an American neurologist who died in 1937. Ramsay Hunt syndrome is a disease of the eighth cranial nerve or the vestibulocochlear nerve. Ramsay Hunt described what happened when the eighth nerve was attacked by the herpes zoster virus, or shingles and he called it Herpes Zoster Oticus (of the ear). There is a vivid rash and blisters along the side of the face, sometimes around the ear, and sometimes extending into the hairline. The person feels increased sensitivity to touch, intense ear pain, hearing loss, vertigo, tinnitus, and sometimes loss of taste, nausea and some accounts mention nystagmus. The rash can be seen around the ear, around the head and face and the person can have a facial palsy.

Ramsay Hunt syndrome is a result of the herpes zoster virus. Subsequent accounts have included other cranial nerves and it seems that the anatomy of the nerves involved in Ramsay Hunt syndrome is more complicated than the usual presentation of shingles which tends to stick to a single nerve.

Andy had many of these symptoms but not the rash. It is possible to have herpes sine zoster, which means the shingles virus without the blisters and rash. It was interesting to read that:-

> The Ramsay Hunt syndrome is associated with brain stem swelling which is 'enhanced' on MRIs of patients with the syndrome, and therefore the medulla is implicated and a link with the nuclei in the brain stem is established.

Ramsay Hunt specifically noticed swelling in the medulla. It was significant that it was increased pressure in the area bounded by the atlas and the axis that appeared to cause Andy's symptoms. It gave some credence to the possibility that mechanical pressure in the medulla could have the same effect on cranial nerves as swelling from infection in the medulla.

If brain stem compression due to infection could cause eighth nerve damage, it could cause damage to the tenth nerve or other nearby cranial nerve nuclei since these nuclei are all close together and on the surface of the medulla. The nuclei of the trigeminal and the facial are also in this vicinity which could provide a link with Gavin's facial pins and needles. It did not, so far, explain Andy's nystagmus.

14 Abducent

Nystagmus, involuntary rhythmic oscillatory movement of the eye, is as complicated as the word suggests. There are several different types of nystagmus, literally 'nodding' eyes which veer towards the side of the semi-circular canals that are being stimulated. There are symmetrical and assymetrical nystagmus, or convergance and retractive nystagmus, mostly congenital or due to disease.

Andy's was a vestibular nystagmus. These are divided into four groups. The first is where there is nystagmus only in one position, usually backwards and rotated called Benign Positional Peripheral Vertigo or BPPV. When nystagmus is found in patients with BPPV it responds to the Hallpike/Epley manoeuvre. Andy did not respond to this as he did not have vertigo due to the position of his head.

There is nystagmus elicited from shaking the head, and nystagmus which occurs at extremes of gaze. The fourth nystagmus is present whatever the position of the head and eyes. This was Andy's nystagmus. It was a straight 'beating' nystagmus that flicked towards his left side, the side where he had all his other symptoms, such as loss of hearing.

Vestibular nystagmus, the literature explains, is due to incorrect messages from the vestibular nuclei to the horizontal gaze centres in the brain. Gray's *Anatomy* revealed which muscle was being irritated in Andy's case.

There are a lot of muscles controlling the eye and each is identified. The muscle that does a sideways (or lateral) movement of the eye, Andy's flickering muscle, is called the rectus lateralis. It has a nerve all to itself. The nerve is the abducent and is the sixth cranial nerve. Control of rectus lateralis of the eye is the only function of the abducent nerve.

If abducent was irritated it could cause flickering of that isolated eye muscle. Where is the abducent in relation to the other, larger, nerve, the one that could already be causing Andy's symptoms, the vestibulocochlear nerve?

A further read of Gray's *Anatomy* reveals that the abducent nerve has a long and tortuous course through the brain. It is therefore vulnerable to the general effects of an increase of pressure from an intracranial mass (tumour, or any other pressure such as mechanical pressure). This pressure may be indirect and not necessarily directly on the nerve itself. The nucleus of abducent is on the floor of the fourth ventricle, and the fourth ventricle is immediately above the area of the medulla.

Any increase in pressure in the medulla which houses the vestibulocochlear and the Vagus would seep upwards to affect the abducent. They are all close enough to be affected by pressure from the atlanto-axial ring. This little gem led one step closer to finding a reason for the labyrinthitis sufferers' symptoms.

15   Virus

"What have you been doing?" Jane asked.

In fairness I should have asked the question first since she had been on an extensive holiday around the east coast of USA, no doubt with misadventures without which no trip taken by Jane seemed complete.

"I have discovered a specific herpes infection of the eighth cranial nerve and I am wondering if there are herpes viruses which affect other cranial nerves."

Jane and I decided to join forces, and while I looked into viruses, Jane agreed to research into herpes.

Viruses are basically parasites, that is, they live in a host, in their case a healthy cell. Some are quite big, like the herpes virus, and some small, like the poliovirus. A virus can pass from person to person in the air, entering the body via the respiratory tract. They can be transmitted from person to person through saliva, kissing or sharing a water bottle — or physical contact including sports like wrestling. Viruses can also be injected by insect bites or infected needles.

The first thing a virus does is attach itself to the surface of a cell. Viruses have a protein shell, a capsid, and an inner core of nucleic acid. The entire particle is called a virion. Some virions have a protective lipid or fatty coat which they wrap around themselves like an envelope. The make-up of the capsid is what makes a specific virus and the core is where the virus is infective. The virion either fuses with the plasma membrane of the host cell or infiltrates it. Capsids are transported towards the nucleus, and its DNA passes into the cell. They do not necessarily kill the host cell in the process.

Because it is a parasite it works inside its host cell and has to work within it. Unfortunately, once the virus is inside the host cell it can infect it, and this cell can infect other cells nearby, by a process called syncytia. When the virus is in the cell it can start replicating, making more identical viruses. So long as the envelope is intact and not damaged, the virus is readily infectious. It can be damaged by alcohol or detergents, such as soap, and made inactive because the solvents work on the fatty envelope.

The effect on the host cell is cytopathic, the virus causes unwanted changes in the cell and the cell undergoes lysis and starts to break down. An infected cell, due to this cytopathic effect, changes. It can become rounded, swollen, shrunken, detached or it can die (apoptosis). The host cell tries to defend itself by apoptosis, but some viruses can delay or prevent apoptosis. Not all virus particles are infectious and it seems that the time they are released depends on the virus and the conditions for it to grow.

The way that the body defends itself is to use the immune system. When measles was rife and there was no vaccine, (it only arrived in 1957), those who survived — and many children did not — built a life-long immunity against further attacks. The measles virus was passed from person to person through the air, and it lodged in the throat and lungs. There the virus incubated and 10-12 days later the person would develop a high fever, with cough, runny nose and sore red eyes. 2-3 days later small spots would appear in the mouth and soon after that a red rash would appear on the face which spread over the entire body. During the four days before and after the appearance of the rash the person was highly infectious.

To prevent viruses such as measles infecting a person a vaccine was developed. Measles has almost been eradicated thanks to a vaccination programme worldwide. Vaccines are harmless agents that are seen by the body as enemies. They are made from live, modified active or dead viruses. Their job is to elicit an immune response which will give the person protection against a particular virus. Each illness, whether measles, mumps or polio, needs its own individual vaccine.

However some viruses mutate. Viruses like the 'flu virus change all the time, and the vaccine does not always work because the changes are in a way that the scientists did not anticipate.

It is not possible to have vaccine for all viruses. The herpes virus for example has no vaccine because there are so many different types and each type has to be targeted separately.

Herpes

	Subfamily	Target Cell Type	Latency	Transmission
1/HSV1	Alpha	mucoepithelial	neuron	close contact
2/HSV2	Alpha	mucoepithelial	neuron	usually sexual
3/VZV	Alpha	mucoepithelial	neuron	contact or respiration
4/EBV	Gamma	epithelial monocytes lymphocytes	b-cells b-cells b-cells	saliva " "
5/CMV	Beta	epithelial monocytes lymphocytes	monocytes and lymphocytes?	contact blood transfusions
6/Herpes Lymphotropic Virus	Beta	T-lymphocytes and others	T-lymphocytes and others	contact respiration
7/HHV7	Beta	"	"	unknown
8/KSHV	Kaposi sarcoma associated Gamma	endothelial	unknown	?Body fluid exchange

16   Richard Hunt

Jane was not very impressed when she saw the paltry amount of notes that I had on viruses. She held up a sheaf of papers. "This is what you sent me to do!"

Jane and I had decided to meet in the Lake District as it was still early in the year, and Jane had found a reasonably priced B&B. However, we had been so intimidated by the many printed notes affixed to the walls, and even in the shower room, with rules as to what we could and could not do, that we had gathered up all our papers and found a table in the wintry sun in a cafe overlooking the lake. "It was the notice four feet from the kitchen door which did it for me," Jane said as we waited for our coffee. "'Do not approach the kitchen beyond this point'. What did they think we were going to do?"

Jane shuffled through her wad of papers. "You won't believe what horrid little creatures herpes are. Not like measles, you know. You have it and that's it, never again. No. Have a little herpes and then it'll hide and come back when you least expect it. They have very nasty habits." Jane was enjoying herself. "Cold sores keep coming back because the virus hides in the nucleus of a nerve."

"There are eight types of herpes. Do you want me to go through them all? I don't need to explain the eighth because that is Kaposi, the AIDS virus." Jane stirred her coffee, took a sip, and then picked up the diagram of the various herpes that affect humans. "There are three groups: alpha, beta and gamma, depending on where the virus lies in wait. The alpha viruses are latent in the Neurons, beta are latent in the T lymphocytes, and the gamma in the B-cells. T-cells are a type of white blood cell that is vital for immunity and comes from the thymus. B-cells are also a type of white blood cell but they work differently in the immune system and they come from bone."

"So the viruses are everywhere? How did you find all this out?"

"I googled 'characteristics of herpes' and eventually found Dr Richard Hunt of South Carolina University. All his work is online for free, which is amazing. So, which shall I tell you about first?"

"Whatever you want."

"The first is Herpes Simplex One or HSV1. It is basically oral herpes. The person has a mild fever and then gets blisters on their mouth, we call them cold sores, or even in their throat. The cold sores are blisters full of virus and it is only when the virus dries up that it dies. The herpes simplex two or genital herpes works in the same way. That is the sexually transmitted herpes."

"What is the difference?"

"One above the waist and the other below. HSV2 just reactivates more efficiently from the lumbo-sacral dorsal root ganglia. If the first viral attack is in the genitalia, then subsequent attacks will be there also."

"What makes a herpes come back?"

"No-one really knows, but there are triggers such as trauma, other infections and stress, which weaken the immune system. Herpes can be triggered by diabetes, influenza, upper respiratory tract infections and pregnancy. There are so many reasons given that one suspects that no one really knows what triggers the virus to reactivate. It may also spread from one ganglia to another."

"Can't doctors stop the virus from coming back?"

"No, they can catch it early when it is active and try to prevent a severe reaction using anti-virals. While it lies dormant there is nothing that can reach it. It is hidden from the immune system."

"So how do they know where it is?" Jane and I sifted through the pages that she had printed out from differing sources.

"They can find it on post-mortem. It is known that herpes prefers sensory nerves and it likes the autonomic system. It chooses cranial nerves and nuclei, autonomic ganglia, and dorsal roots near the spine. Each time an outbreak of herpes clears up, it leaves no trace, no scars, and the person recovers completely. There are complications, however, from both HSV1 and HSV2 that include inflammation of the brain coverings, tonsillitis and sore throat, inflammation of the lungs, and, HSV2 can be passed to the unborn child."

Before moving on to Human Herpes Virus 3, HHV3, we packed our files into our useful little backpacks and, following a trail around the lake, walked until we reached another café. We were, after all, physiotherapists who spend our working lives encouraging exercise and we could hardly allow ourselves to sit around all morning.

17   Herpes Zoster

"If that is herpes simplex, what is a complicated herpes like?"

"HHV3 is Varicella Zoster Virus or VZV. VZV includes both chicken pox and shingles." Jane was being deliberately confusing. Then she relented. "Chickenpox is becoming less common but it is a highly contagious airborne virus, the varicella virus. In children, who, often, do not have the low fever or nausea or aching muscles that adults experience, it starts with a rash or spots in the mouth that then appear all over the torso of the body. The bumps become pustules and blisters, and then they finally scab over. The incubation period is 14-21 days. The person is contagious until the blisters have crusted over. You get it from close skin or saliva contact. That is as far as varicella goes to resembling a regular virus. What happens next is that the virus disappears up a nerve and becomes latent and lies dormant in a nerve cell. Later, sometimes years and years later, the virus will reactivate and travel back down the axon to cause a viral infection in the skin in the region of the nerve and once again there will be a rash, and then the person develops shingles."

"How does shingles start?"

"Herpes Zoster starts with a low grade malaise and it is often only when the rash appears that the diagnosis is made. Shingles differs from chickenpox in that the skin lesions are small and close together and are along the pathway of a nerve. It causes a painful rash which usually heals in two to four weeks but the pain can last for a very long time afterwards. Sometimes the rash is in areas of skin far afield from the location of the latent virus. Only half of shingles patients actually have the rash and there are more cases of complications of the nervous system than were previously acknowledged. Shingles has to be diagnosed within three days for anti-virals such as acyclovir or valaclovir to work. Shingles can come back again and again. Sometimes recurrences are as often as every 14 -21 days."

"Where can you have shingles?" I asked.

"Almost anywhere in the body. If the virus stays moist then it can remain active. It can also evade the immune system so that it is hard to destroy. The virus can escape the immune system by coating itself with immunoglobulin. This means that a person's own cells have to fight the virus using Natural Killer Cells, or cause an inflammatory reaction such as fever to control the infection by producing a substance called interferon."

Jane then surprised me. "I have been thinking. Do you think that Andy had Ramsay Hunt syndrome? Do you think that his labyrinthitis could have been caused by an infection not of his labyrinths but of his vestibulocochlear nerve?"

Andy's labyrinthitis had had a sudden onset and he had felt ill subsequently for weeks, unlike the other cases. He had specifically reported that 'he had felt brilliant that morning', on the day that he had had to call the ambulance, which was an unusual observation, but a heightened sense of wellbeing can precede a systemic infection.

"You mean herpes without the spots, herpes sine zoster? Now you suggest it, I think that you might be right. It would explain why some of his symptoms cleared up and some like his deafness and nystagmus did not. There could be permanent damage if it had been an infection. That might explain why only some of his problems were cleared up due to treatment at the atlanto-axial joint."

Jane nodded for me to go on. "We might have to start re-thinking what might be the reasons behind the labyrinthitis cases and how each cranial nerve might be implicated. I think that Lois and Angie had labyrinthitis due to the atlanto-axial joint because in both cases all of their symptoms cleared up and physiotherapy was the only intervention."

"So that leaves Gavin."

"He is still a puzzle."

"You know that herpes means 'creep'." Jane announced.

"As in, you little creep, or as in creeping ivy?"

"No idea, it's Greek. Both I suspect."

The Lakes have a café around every corner, and we were soon ensconced at a table as far from other holiday makers as possible. We were aware that we looked too earnest and that our bookishness was a bit embarrassing but it was difficult to be inconspicuous because Jane's attire was hardly subdued. Jane has a reputation for slightly bohemian and very colourful clothing. My attire, of course, was the epitome of the discreet, bordering on the drab.

"The fourth herpes is EBV or Epstein-Barr Virus."

"Glandular fever is a herpes?" I asked, incredulous.

"Herpes is the second most common form of illness after 'flu and the common cold." Jane explained. "With glandular fever the person has a high fever for 10-14 days, sore throat, fatigue, swollen glands and aching muscles which last about three weeks. The person has small red spots in their throat, enlarged tonsils and sometimes a rash. The virus replicates in epithelial cells which line our mouths and throat, and then later lies dormant in the B-cells in the blood. It is transmitted by saliva and has a long incubation period of 4-6 weeks. The person can be infectious for ages afterwards but because it has low infectivity it is not passed on to many people."

"That's the kissing disease! What is this next one? Cytomegalovirus?" I find it impossible not to be intrigued by long medical names. "Cyto.Cells. Mega. Big?"

"CMV. This one is a bit like having EBV but this is a Beta herpes and it lies dormant in the monocytes and lymphocytes which are types of white blood cells. It is passed from person to person via most secretions but in hospitals through blood transfusion. It is caused by infection in the salivary glands, testes, kidneys and the cervix. The sad thing is that it can be passed from a mother to her baby before it is born." Jane showed me a print out. The poor child was covered in a violent red rash. "CMV reappears particularly when a person's immune system is down, and weirdly, the virus itself can cause the immune system to be stressed."

"So the virus itself can be the reason for another virus to attack?"

"Yes." Jane shivered. "My hands are getting really cold." Everyone at the other tables had disappeared, but Jane was ready to talk about the next herpes.

"HHV6. This is another Beta. It doesn't cause cold sores or blisters and almost everyone is affected by HHV6 by the time they are two. It causes a rash in children, on their faces, and fever and diarrhoea. The virus comes back in all sorts of areas of the body, like the heart, brain, lungs, or gut. It is thought that it could have something to do with other illnesses such as multiple sclerosis, epilepsy and chronic fatigue syndrome."

"CFS? Really?"

"HHV6 can remain in the central nervous system long after it has disappeared from the blood stream. In 2012 patients with CFS who were treated with long-term anti-virals such as valganciclovir had good results and 81% improved cognitive function. Another CFS group studied showed 75% improvement and continued improvement over 2-3 years."

"Oh!" I said, as we relocated to a table inside the café where a log fire was burning. "We never got onto number seven."

"It was bunched into the same category as number six." Jane explained. "I didn't mention it because not an awful lot is known. It infects children between ages of three and five, after they've had HHV6!"

"It's strange that it should have a number all to itself!" I commented.

"One day it might be the magic number and hold the key to unravelling some of the illnesses that still are unexplained."

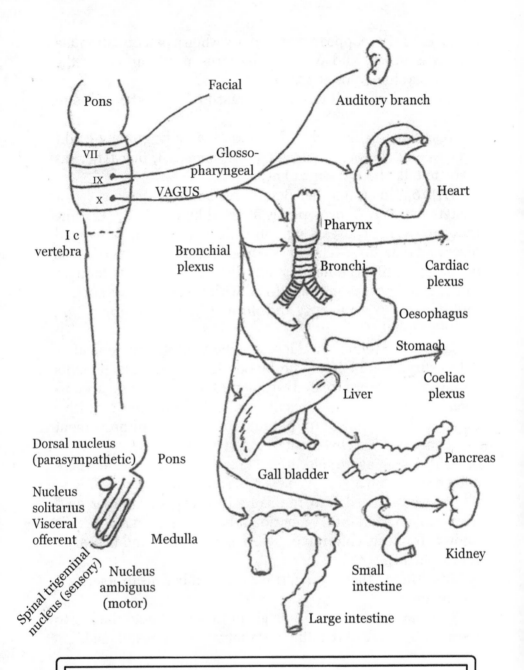

Pons

VII

IX

X

I c
vertebra

Facial

Glosso-
pharyngeal

VAGUS

Auditory branch

Heart

Pharynx

Bronchial
plexus

Bronchi

Cardiac
plexus

Oesophagus

Stomach

Coeliac
plexus

Liver

Dorsal nucleus
(parasympathetic)

Pons

Nucleus
solitarius
Visceral
offerent

Medulla

Spinal trigeminal
nucleus (sensory)

Nucleus
ambiguus
(motor)

Gall bladder

Pancreas

Kidney

Small
intestine

Large intestine

Parasympathetic nerves

Parasympathetic cranial nerves in the medulla.

19   Parasympathetic

Lois and I were meeting for another Spanish session. We were both a bit rusty. When she had returned from USA Lois admitted that while she was on holiday she had abandoned her *espanol*, and I reassured her by saying that I had ditched the present subjunctive of *haber* in favour of the atlas.

"Mi hermano se siente maravilloso."

"¿Qué?" I answered, rather like a certain Italian waiter.

"My brother! His back has never felt better and his energy has returned. He's been working for ten hours a day. He has even been doing his calf exercises." Lois had been on the telephone to Gavin.

"He told me that his calves felt tight. The acupuncturist had remarked that Gavin's body was waterlogged and I assumed that it was due to the leukaemia." I went on to explain as much to myself as to Lois. "However, if his body could drain better some of his symptoms might reduce. If everything was stuck in the bottle neck at the atlas then his head could not drain. Once the neck area is less congested then the nerves can free up. That is how I imagine it might work. Still, I am glad."

Although Lois knew about the Vagus I was not sure if I had explained about the parasympathetic, the 'rest and digest' portion of the autonomic system.

The parasympathetic includes the third cranial nerve, the oculomotor; the seventh, the facial; the ninth, the glossopharyngeal; as well as the tenth, the Vagus. The oculomotor controls the pupil sphincter muscles and ciliary body which controls the shape of the lens of the eye, the facial controls the lacrimal or tear, nasal and maxillary glands, and the glosspharyngeal controls the parotid gland.

"If the Vagus was being irritated then the parasympathetic nervous system would be activated. Possibly Gavin's increase in energy was due to a release in pressure on his Vagus." The Vagus, as Twink had pointed out, was the arch regulator of the parasympathetic nervous system.

I said that this was what we needed to look at next. "If the parasympathetic was disrupted from its usual function the result would be to exaggerate the functions of the organs that it supplies."

Lois looked doubtful. "And that means?" she asked.

"Everything the Vagus is meant to do, it would do to excess."

"Is that why Gavin and I felt tired?" Prompted Lois.

"Well for one thing muscles take longer to recover. Patients with autonomic disorders have low levels of oxygen uptake, and poor cardio-vascular response during exercise. Muscles have difficulty in taking up oxygen, including the heart, because it is also a muscle."

I read from the study I had on hand.

" 'Exercise increases vagal tone which means that, in people whose Vagus has already slowed down, the effects of exercise would be detrimental. Exercise has the effect of decreasing the sympathetic and so the usual channel of stimulating an organ or a system, is not employed.'"

"Okay, I'll take your word for it! What else do you have?" She asked.

"One of the other effects of a disrupted autonomic system are changes to sweating patterns. In fact your brother has some of these problems. There is hyperhidrosis which is too much sweating or anidrosis, too little, or gustatory sweating which is sweating after meals. Then there is hypothermia or hyperpyrexia which is feeling inappropriately cold or hot." I read on. "In the gut there would be alimentary problems with xerostomia which is a dry mouth, which Gavin complained of, and gastric stasis with the food not passing through the gut properly and getting stuck."

Lois looked suitably impressed.

Later I rang Jane and asked her what might be the reasons behind the various symptoms experienced by the labyrinthitis sufferers.

Jane suggested that the orthostatic intolerance and associated light-headedness were caused by blood pooling into the viscera and leaving the brain. This central pooling, which preserves the integrity of the vital organs, would also account for the pallor and reduced temperature of the extremities which is seen in the face, hands and feet.

If sweating is activated by acetylcholine, which is a sympathetic response to a crisis, and the parasympathetic is sensitive to acetylcholine, this might account for the excessive amount of sweat that people experience in response, for example, to an infection.

On the subject of feeling tired, Jane pointed out that if the pancreas produced too much insulin, then the person would become low in sugar, such as when a diabetic has a 'hypo' episode. If they are low in sugar they would feel low in energy.

Tiredness would also be produced from poor sleep. Sleep is regulated by the parasympathetic and it is necessary for healing and repair.

Finally we discussed flushes and palpitations.

Jane knew what she was talking about where these symptoms were concerned. "Isn't that something to do with the sympathetic trying to correct the situation, like a sympathetic upsurge?" It would be the body trying to counteract an up-regulated parasympathetic. This reminded me of an unusual case that I had been treating for a few weeks.

"Did I tell you about Letty?" I asked. "Her main problems following a car crash were hot flushes and an increased heart rate. It looks as if the sympathetic is in overdrive but it could be reacting to counter the effect of a parasympathetic that has gone crazy."

Letty had presented with the most curious symptoms following her whiplash injury.

20 Letty

Letty had been travelling as a passenger in the front seat of their car when they lost control on black ice. The collision was sufficient to knock down a telegraph pole and the air bags inflated. Thinking that the dust was smoke, Letty got out of the car as fast as possible, but finding herself trapped in a ditch she climbed back through the car, and was helped out of the driver's side by her husband who pulled her by her arms. All passengers appeared to be unharmed.

The next morning Letty was unable to get out of bed. She had vertigo and felt as if the bed and the whole room were moving around her. This stopped when she finally stood, but any movement of her head backward or to the left caused vertigo. Her vertigo has persisted.

Whenever she has an attack of vertigo, which happens with every unguarded movement, her colour rises and her face is flushed and she becomes sweaty with clammy hands and feet, feels anxious and 'spaced out' and her heart rate increases. These episodes could last several hours.

Since the accident Letty has had joint problems, a permanent buzzing, tinnitus and loss of some hearing in her left ear, pins and needles intermittently down her left arm and on the left side of her face, and generalised pain across her shoulders. Her balance problems were severe. She was unable to lie flat and slept in a chair reclined to fifteen degrees from upright. Her cognitive ability had not been affected and she was not down-hearted more than would be expected from such limitations to her life.

A severe assault at work in 1982 when she was in her early forties damaged Letty's neck and abdomen and had left her with abdominal adhesions and a lifetime of digestive problems. She had her appendix removed at that time due to a carcinoid tumour. She was back at work fourteen weeks later.

Letty noticed that her balance was less good about three years ago. She walked with a slightly 'wooden' gait but managed when walking forwards. If she stepped sideways, especially to the right, her symptoms returned and took about four minutes to settle. The hot flushes were instantaneous following any head movement but she was not inhibited by pain.

Letty has had two injuries now to her neck. The first left her with mild problems but the injury was severe. The second 'whiplash' appears to have been the precipitator of the majority of her present, severely handicapping, symptoms.

The flushes and loss of balance, and 'scared' feeling are indicative of autonomic disturbance. The pins and needles down her left arm and weakness in both shoulder muscles as well as a heightened sensitivity to touch throughout her body were musculo-skeletal signs of neurological damage from spinal nerves.

Whiplash injury at the atlanto-axial joint compressing the Vagus nerve and triggering the parasympathetic could give Letty her feelings of disorientation, anxiety and loss of balance. The manner in which Letty's body responds to the triggering of the parasympathetic is by using the sympathetic, the characteristic signs of which are racing heart, rush of blood to the face, brain and periphery, and a closing down of the internal organs. It seems that the mechanism operating is too much sympathetic activity. The doctor had tried to help with medication for the sympathetic activity but it had not been successful possibly because the symptoms were not systemically mediated. The doctor had always maintained that the whiplash had triggered Letty's vertigo.

The treatment plan for Letty was the reverse to that undertaken in the other four cases of vertigo. Assessing or treating her atlanto-axial joint was out of the question because even a slight pressure on her skull produced vertigo for over five minutes. Due to the heightened sensitivity of all of Letty's tissues, in her first treatment she only managed five minutes of gentle massage to her feet before her body had a sympathetic reaction.

It was soon obvious that tackling Letty's vertigo was going to be a very long process. With some misgivings I warned her about the length of time we were looking at if we were to have any hope of unpicking her symptoms.

"It could take up to a year." I said.

Her response was not one that I anticipated. "That gives me such relief." She assured me. "I feared that you might think that we had to hurry, and I know myself that this will take time."

In fact, although it took some three months before we had any consistent progress with her treatment, the small incremental inroads into de-sensitising her body slowly paid off. After six months Letty could tolerate fascia work to her forearms and lower limbs and gentle mobilisation to her lumbar spine while sitting with no back support with barely a reaction. At this point she was able, at different times during the week, to rest her feet on a vibrating board, roll and squeeze a soft ball in her hands, stand on a two centimetre high board and drop her heels, walk with arm swing for 800 yards, complete breathing exercises that included all three dimensions, use a sitting pedal machine for three to five minutes, and sit to stand without feeling dizzy.

What she could not do was infinite, but her most inconveniencing problems were drying herself after a shower, leaning forward for example to play cards, turn her head in any direction, or, most importantly, lie down.

21   Alpha Beta Gamma

"¡Buenas tardes, Amiga!"

"¡Bienvenido!"

"Antes la clase…" Lois began. She asked if, before we started, we could discuss the labyrinth story so far. "The atlas and the axis, how do they move?"

"There are three boney rings, the occiput, the atlas and the axis. Each bone is joined by ligaments which work like tough rubber rings. These allow the joints to move by sliding, sheering and rotating. Into the central hole fits the stalk of the brain, a bundle of nervous tissue, which becomes the spinal cord. When you moved your head," I demonstrated to Lois with my hands, "the boney rings did not move efficiently and this squashed the nervous tissue so that it could not conduct messages correctly. What you were squashing were the nuclei or the power houses of the nerves."

"I understand that these nuclei are beside the atlas and the axis in the medulla. I can see that each nerve has a separate purpose and each can give a reason for some of the things we are telling you about in our physiotherapy treatments. Are you suggesting that the Ramsay Hunt syndrome is an infection of the eighth cranial nerve and from it you can get symptoms like Andy's?"

"Yes. Both an infection and pressure from joints can impact on a nucleus."

"So pressure on the seventh could cause pins and needles in Gavin's face?"

"That is a bit more complicated. The facial is motor to the face. If it is damaged you would see a Bell's Palsy, a dropped face, but the nerve links with the trigeminal, and this is sensory to the face. The fact that he has pins and needles on both sides of his face means that the problem has to be central. That means it has to be in the medulla. Bell's Palsy is only ever on one side."

"The sixth, the abducent, does the flickering eye!" Lois said, pleased with herself.

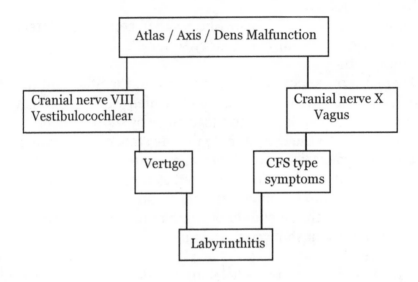

Mechanical malfunction of the dens simultaneously affects vestibulocochlear and Vagus nuclei. The vestibulocochlear causes symptoms of vertigo and the Vagus causes Chronic Fatigue Syndrome-like symptoms. The combination results in Labyrinthitis.

"And the ninth, the glossopharyngeal seems to cover the mouth and throat symptoms."

Lois then said. "Jane seems to think that the Vagus is important because it is parasympathetic. Is that because the weird symptoms, like loss of energy, are due to the Vagus? Is the tenth the one that could be causing all of our psychological problems?" Lois said this with a knowing smile; she was not a psychotherapist for nothing.

"That is where the journey has got to now. Those symptoms could be parasympathetic symptoms and explain your horrid feelings, but we would have to find a disease caused by an infected Vagus, like the Ramsay Hunt, to see what really happens."

We had to find if there were any illnesses that were due to infection of the Vagus.

If a similar scenario could be found for the Vagus, in other words an infection of its nucleus which caused an illness whose symptoms corresponded to those experienced by the labyrinth patients, then we could be in a position to say that Lois's labyrinth symptoms were due to mechanical pressure of the Vagus.

We had to find this elusive illness.

That evening I contacted Jane.

"Which of all these herpes is most likely to annoy the Vagus?" I asked.

"Well, if it is a neurone we are looking at it has to be an Alpha," Jane replied. It sounded as if we were choosing hats. 'If it is for the Artic then I suggest this one.'

"The Alpha herpes are cold sores, genital herpes and varicella or herpes zoster, basically the first three."

"And the fourth is a Beta?" I asked.

"No EBV is a Gamma. It lies dormant in the blood in b-cells. The Beta herpes are five, six and seven which are in different blood cells. However they all like mucous linings, and although they transmit in different ways, they all lie dormant somewhere. They all multiply and then shed when they feel like it, but particularly when the person is stressed. Sometimes stressed by a low immune system due to another virus."

"And that virus could also be a herpes?"

"Yes."

It was becoming more complicated, not less, but Jane had given warning.

"And all herpes clear up. Usually by drying out." Jane continued. "The difference with the Vagus is that it is internal and so, unlike herpes that migrate to the skin, healing from an internal herpes is more difficult."

"So you can get herpes inside the body?"

"Yes, that is where the complications occur, and they are often pretty serious."

"What do you mean?"

"Meningitis and other brain tissue infections, pneumonias in the lungs, or infections in the heart or liver."

"How would it get there?" I wondered.

"Like any other herpes, from the outside, and lodge in the mucous linings. Then the virus can track up a nerve and later transfer to another nerve if it wants."

"There seem to be several ways that a person can catch herpes."

"Herpes are transmitted by different routes. All herpes can be transmitted by close contact and all herpes enter the body through some mucous lining whether it be via the mouth, throat, respiratory passages or the genitalia. What is more herpes is 'endemic', it is around all the time."

I felt a little more knowledgeable when Lois and I next met up. Lois had another set of questions ready.

"Why do people get herpes?" Lois asked.

"If it is chickenpox they can catch it if they have not already had it. It is highly contagious. HSV2 is catching as is EBV, but these differ because not everyone gets sick from catching them. Then there are the herpes that arrive second time around so to speak. They have been there all the time lying dormant and then one decides to activate and shed its virus making the person ill, like getting shingles. They can all return again giving the person sporadic episodes when they become ill."

"What does the herpes virus do?"

"It causes a specific illness the first time around, like glandular fever. The next time the herpes causes an illness it is less specific. There is a low grade fever, sore throat, headache, malaise or feeling ill, perhaps a rash, swollen or tender lymph nodes."

"Does anything show on tests?" Lois asked hopefully.

I could only disappoint her. "The inflammation interferes with natural cell death and causes oxidative stress, but as the virus is only active for a short while often nothing is seen on blood tests. Herpes can evade the immune system. There is no method yet of finding the latent virus." Then I remembered something else that Jane had ferreted out. "What they do know is that herpes likes sensory nerves, and it especially likes the parasympathetic nerves"

"The illness that herpes gives is really just like any 'bug.'" Lois summarised.

"Yes, but don't forget that people completely recover from herpes."

"Always?"

"Unless they get complications. I know that sounds a bit contradictory, but when people recover they recover completely for instance from cold sores, chickenpox, glandular fever and eventually from the others even if they return episodically."

In the following few days I trawled through the literature Jane had sent me to research illnesses of the Vagus nerve and to find out how a deranged Vagus nerve affected people, but there was little to find. However, I had a reasonably clear idea where the trail could be leading. When we met for our next session of Spanish, Lois said.

"At one point during my spell of labyrinthitis, I could understand my vertigo and nausea being due to my balance mechanisms, but I could not understand why I felt so awful, so lacking in energy, anxious and with brain fog. I thought that I had ME."

I suspected that Jane too had come to the same conclusion, and when I rang her she confirmed this.

This was not as extraordinary as it seems. All three of us had an unusual and unpleasant history in common. Lois had a daughter and Jane and I both had a son with CFS/ME or Chronic Fatigue Syndrome/ Myalgic Encephalomyelitis.

However much we all sensed that this was a possible answer, all effects of CFS/ME would have to be explained by infection of the Vagus. If in Ramsay Hunt syndrome herpes was able to affect the vestibulocochlear, herpes could just as easily affect the Vagus. Was it possible that infection of the Vagus nerve had common ground with CFS/ME?

Lois had her customary index cards with her. Every week she would produce her recent Spanish language finds. There might be a new expression; 'fuero lo que fuese' for 'whatever it was', or 'de todos modos' for 'all the same'. Her favourites were false friends; 'sensible' meaning 'sensitive', 'exito' meaning 'success' or 'constipado' meaning ' a bad cold'.

"CFS is a false friend." Lois announced.

"How do you mean?" I asked.

"Well, it makes people think they know what it is, but the majority of people don't."

"Would you jot down what it really is like? Jane and I can do the medical translation to see how it might fit with the Vagus."

The next day Lois dropped two index cards through my letterbox.

The first read:

This is what ME people say about their illness.

I feel tired all the time. I can't go to school. What I am reading does not make sense. I have a headache. The light hurts my eyes. Please close the curtains. Please don't drive so fast. I can't go into that shop. The smell is too strong. I want to play games. I want to go for a walk. If I go for a walk I will not be able to do anything tomorrow.

When I stand up I feel dizzy. Please don't let my friend stay too long. I can't talk much. Please turn down the TV. I can only watch easy films. I am cold all the time. I need an electric toothbrush. My heart goes funny sometimes. That yogurt smells off. My legs twitch and are restless all the time. My stomach hurts. I can't sleep. I can only sleep for five hours. I cannot get to sleep. Often I am awake all night.

This was not at all what I expected but it portrayed ME much more vividly than any list.

The second card was equally unusual:

This is what other people say to ME patients.

You look pale. You had better lie down. Can I cut it up for you? What do you think you can eat? Do you want a painkiller? Why are you not wearing shoes? Why are you not wearing a watch? Why are you using plastic cutlery? Do you think you can walk a hundred yards, wouldn't it do you good? Why don't you get up earlier and then you would sleep. Why are you bolshie? Why don't you have a warm drink and a bath each night and go to bed in good time. Try this book. Try this puzzle. Why could you do that yesterday and not to-day? Why don't you try some homework? Fresh air might help, you would not look so pale.

"What does CFS/ME have in common with labyrinthitis? What else do we know about CFS/ME?" Lois's question was almost rhetorical because we had both read Dr Melvin Ramsay's 'Saga'.

Dr Melvin Ramsay had been the doctor who named ME and he had seen and was the first to report what the illness was like when there was an outbreak in a London hospital in 1955.

Early symptoms are malaise and headache. Frequent disproportionate depression and emotional lability/ fluctuations. This might disappear for a day or two and then return more severely, with mild sore throat, severe headache of a new kind and nausea/ feeling sick with anorexia/not wanting to eat, sometimes abdominal pain, vomiting and diarrhoea. In some cases the full picture did not develop for 2-3weeks.

Then pain in the neck and back or limbs, or below the rib margins would develop. Patients became more ill at this stage and there was central nervous system involvement in three-quarters of the patients. Many varied signs were observed:

Cranial nerves, blurring vision, tinnitus, nystagmus and some facial problems;

Weak trunk muscles, painful twitches and some with bladder dysfunction;

Pain and marked muscular tenderness and tingling in muscles. Always; muscles fatigued easily.

Other signs found were orthostatic intolerance with rapid heart rate; ghastly facial pallor; coldness of extremities.

Cognitive symptoms were: memory, concentration and emotional impairment; vivid dreams; sensitivity to sound.

Sleep disorders. Changed behaviour in children.

Observed were: tender lymph nodes and glands; stiff neck; sore throat; vesicles in throat. And 20% had a recurrence within a year.

"We seem to heading away from labyrinthitis." Lois ventured.

"Into unchartered waters" I added for her. "Not totally, only for a while, because we can't argue the reasons for labyrinthitis without finding an illness for the Vagus."

"But everyone says that no-one knows what ME is." Lois objected.

"That's true, but an awful lot *is* known about ME." I countered.

Lois was thoughtful. "Although the sore throat type bug is the same for ME and lots of other illnesses, there are similarities with herpes aren't there? You know, the way it keeps coming back." Lois was thinking of her daughter.

"But," I said, trying to be a little more optimistic, "both herpes and ME can clear up completely, and that can't be said of most cases of diseases of the nervous system."

"So what do we do now?" Lois asked, reasonably enough.

"Now we have to look at what is already known about ME and what we know about the Vagus. And then see if the jigsaw fits."

"And a possible infection?"

"Herpes?"

Dr Melvin Ramsay used a photograph of a herpes in its envelope as the illustration on the front cover of his book which he published in 1986. He wrote:

The future will probably relate to persistent virus infections and in this group are included many of the herpes group of viruses.

CFS/ME can have a sudden or a gradual onset and every ME patient can tell you *when* their CFS/ME started. Dr Melvin Ramsay said that three signs were present in *every* case of ME. These are muscle fatigability where even after a minor degree of effort up to four or five days may be needed before the muscle regains full power; circulatory impairment where the person has cold extremities and whose face often goes an ashen grey colour; and cognitive dysfunction where memory, concentration and emotional instability are features.

Jane's son was diagnosed for months with high blood pressure and then a virus precipitated his illness. My son had been slowly finding school more and more difficult before being ill for three years. Lois's daughter had succumbed after a short 'bug' from which she did not recover for months and has had three bad bouts over nine years

Was the illness pattern of ME compatible with what is known of the illness process of herpes?

One aspect that both herpes and ME have in common is that there are outbreaks or epidemics. A chickenpox outbreak is an example of an epidemic of a herpes illness. Fifty-two outbreaks of CFS/ME have been recorded throughout the world since 1934. The most recent outbreak in UK was in West Kilbride and Balfron in Scotland where there were thirty-eight cases in 1984.

The largest outbreak of ME, as it went on to be called, was in the Royal Free hospital where Dr Melvin Ramsay was the physician in charge of infectious diseases. 292 members of the medical and other hospital workers were affected by the illness, as were 12 of the patients who were in hospital at the time.

Both herpes, after the initial illness, and ME are difficult to detect on testing. In ME all tests come back negative because ME is usually not diagnosed until the patient has been unwell for six months or more, and any viral activity is no longer evident.

Herpes and ME are known to be endemic, in other words they crop up regularly in isolated incidents. The Epstein-Barr virus is an example. Many students can test positive for EBV but only the odd student will actually develop glandular fever/mononucleosis.

Both herpes and ME are believed to be triggered by many of the same factors and each initial illness begins with a high fever. Like herpes sufferers the majority of people who have ME already have a weak immune system due to physical or emotional trauma, vaccinations or previous infection such as glandular fever.

A pattern of an initial illness followed by relapses and remissions is a characteristic of herpes and ME. A pattern of complete recovery in most cases is also common to both.

Herpes is usually associated with a rash and some CFS/ME patients do at some point have a rash. Onsets of herpes such as HHV1, HHV3 and HHV4 commence with a sore throat and Dr Melvin Ramsay noticed vesicles in the throats of some of the Royal Free patients.

ME is an illness where longevity is the rule. HSV2 is also known to persist for months or years. There is no known cause for ME and similarly there is no known reason why viruses reactivate.

It is particularly hard for people living with undiagnosed conditions or those who are given labels such as labyrinthitis or chronic fatigue which fundamentally mean unexplained symptoms. The effect of not knowing why they are ill on the lives of labyrinthitis and CFS/ME patients can be compared, without too much exaggeration, to what the Bosnian concentration camp victims had to endure when under siege and afterwards.

Patients will tell you that they can face anything if they know the reason for their illness and what can be done about it. It is the 'not knowing' that is the stumbling block. In Sarajevo the Bosnians knew their adversaries, and could do something to avoid them, they knew who their killers were and when they were vulnerable. Every time that it was possible to see a hillside from a street, and Sarajevo is surrounded by hills, the citizens were at risk of sniper fire. Buses were stationed so as to guard thoroughfares and provide protection. Holes were drilled from house to house to make safe passages. On the hillsides Serbians who used to be neighbours would taunt the inhabitants, sometimes by name, before setting off sniper fire. They had some control.

Those who suffered most during the war were those in the concentration camps, often isolated high rise flats rather than the more familiar barb wire enclosures, not knowing when the next assault would be perpetrated. Once the war was over there was additional anxiety for the women whose men had not returned and whose graves had not been found. There was no aid available until the bodies had been identified. Some had still not been found even ten years later.

In medicine, however dire the diagnosis, any patient will tell you that being in limbo during investigations or awaiting an operation, is worse than the event itself. Patients with CFS/ME and labyrinthitis who have no timescale for their illness nor effective treatment are, like the women waiting for news, in limbo. Like their Bosnian counterparts they are stuck in a life where they have to endure their condition with no obvious end in sight. This was why Jane and I went to Sarajevo. This is why Lois's case of labyrinthitis, and our children's cases of ME, became an obsession. This is why the enigma of labyrinthitis and CFS/ME urgently needs to be solved.

Yet emotion has no place in serious scientific study and just as I was fearing that the Vagus nerve theory was relying on only a few cases and therefore was likely to have little credibility, Lois hit her head.

This incident, occurring as it did some nine months after she had recovered from her vertigo, although conveniently timed for this story, was devastating for her. A storm had caused a power cut and, in the dark, Lois had slipped and fallen. She heard a crack in her skull as she fell. She also injured her right elbow. Subsequently, although no area of her skull was sore to touch, she had a headache in the left parietal-occipital region. Lois went for a check-up with her GP but she had not been concussed.

Four weeks after the accident Lois woke with vertigo and nausea, and, in a panic, made an appointment for the afternoon which was, fortunately, a day for Spanish.

When I saw her, Lois explained that her vertigo was mild but hovering. She still had all her other symptoms, was unable to run and could only walk slowly up and down stairs or hills. Her mind was clear which was a relief, especially since we were tackling the tricky conundrum as to when the Spanish use the perfect and when the present indicative. (The answer is that it depends on how it relates to the present moment). At the present moment all that Lois cared about was not slipping into another bout of labyrinthitis.

The movements of her neck that were most restricted were extension and rotation to the left. Every movement of her neck elicited soreness on the left side, mainly around the fourth cervical vertebra, and at the base of her cranium. I treated all the areas of the cranium and mobilised her neck at the relevant joints.

One day later Lois reported that her head and neck were pretty sore but that her vertigo and nausea had cleared.

A week later Lois returned. She had no dizziness and her gut had settled — she said that the two usually went together — but that she still had the neck and lower sacro-iliac back pain. Her headache had disappeared two days previously.

24   Breakthrough

Jane decided to travel north for a visit. It seemed only logical to invite Lois over. The unravelling of the vertigo conundrum was a common factor which would act as an ice breaker.

Not that ice breakers are really needed where Jane is concerned. "Hello, Labyrinth Lois!" Jane called out as Lois entered the kitchen. Long gone were the days when she had to ring the doorbell.

Lois responded with, "Holá! Amigas!" which nicely levelled their opening gambits.

We settled around the kitchen table where I had a small pile of recent copies of the ME Research journal *Breakthrough*. I explained that we needed the established facts about CFS/ME and that each edition contained a world overview of current research. Picking one out at random I handed it to Jane.

I picked up a second copy while Lois browsed through a third.

"I'll write and you read." Lois suggested.

"Listen to this! Not a wonder CFS/ME people complain about their eyes. Twenty-five per cent have to give up driving."

"Why?" Asked Lois conscientiously starting to write.

"Their eyes give out. The muscles fatigue and they cannot focus. They get distracted by irrelevant material and cannot scan or follow a target on screen. Their eyes cannot move smoothly. Basically this affects their ability to read, and to cope with bright lights."

"Photophobia." said Lois knowledgeably. When you have lived alongside ME for years you begin to pick up these terms.

"I have one on muscles." Jane said. "They were looking for an easy test to show how muscles fatigue. They gave CFS/ME people a dynamometer."

"Dynamometer?"

"It's a rubber bulb that you grip and then squeeze and it has a dial indicating strength in pounds. Each person in the study squeezed the dynamometer eighteen times. The healthy people could repeat the test immediately with no loss of strength, but the CFS/ME people even after thirty or forty minutes rest could not reach the same poundage."

There was a spell of quiet while Jane and I scanned further articles.

"HHV6 might be important because of how it reacts with other viruses to muck up the immune function. So one virus can set another off, just as Dr Melvin Ramsay thought that the polio virus might have done in 1955." I read.

"Here's one about the heart." Jane had spent many years working with heart patients and was naturally drawn to that subject. "Resting pressure of the heart during diastole, which is while the heart is relaxing between beats, is lower, and this gives a lower flow of blood to the muscles and to the brain."

"Is there anything else about the brain?" Lois asked.

I searched my journal. "There is one about sleep. Brains need sleep to clear toxins."

"Every ME person has sleep problems."

"Yes, it says here 97% of ME patients have sleep problems. Scientists say that this could lead to degeneration of the nervous tissue and be the cause of brain fog. Also of memory problems, concentration and information processing."

"That is why they feel stupid at times." Lois commented.

"On PET scans there is widespread inflammation of the brain and in all sorts of different areas and the different areas corresponded with the severity of particular symptoms." I skimmed down the report. "Scientists suggest that it may be due to an immune response to an underlying infectious process."

Jane took up a second journal. "This will interest the physios among us. Nerve stretches. They are really tight, especially in young people."

"I found that in all the labyrinth cases. Do you remember, Lois, when I stretched your arms out to test your nerves?" Lois was not sure. "I found it on slump, upper and lower limb testing with Gavin and Andy."

"Whether the nerves were squeezed due to the joints or due to an infection causing swelling, any thickening in the medulla would restrict nerve movement wouldn't it?" Jane reasoned.

I held up my next article and gave a bit of a laugh. "The parasympathetic again! The study compared 50 to 70 year olds with 25 to 29 year olds. They had had CFS/ME for an average of 92 months. It says that the effects are worse the older you are."

"What effects do they mention?" Jane asked.

"Parasympathetic symptoms such as more fatigue, more depression and poorer quality of life. That's depressing in itself." I remarked.

"Rituximab!" We all knew about the trial that had taken place in Norway of this chemotherapy drug. The first trial had been remarkably successful in treating CFS patients.

"Rituximab works by targeting the B-cells."

"B-cells," repeated Jane, "Epstein Barr Virus is latent in the B-cells. That might be significant."

"Anyway they are doing a larger trial, and aiming to do a similar one in London." I hoped that this was cheering news for Lois. Indeed for all three of us as no-one can be complacent about ME because of its propensity to recur.

Jane seemed a bit preoccupied, and so I pointed out another report to Lois.

"This may not be as far-fetched as it seems." I commented. " 'A link with the Vagus and depression and anxiety. For about seven years now treatment for depression has included an alternative to medication. Originally used for epilepsy, stimulation of the Vagus nerve using a pacemaker has now been pioneered for the relief of depression. The electrical pacemaker is implanted into the chest wall, and the stimulator is targeted towards the left Vagus nerve in the neck. It seems that after a few months the person's depression begins to lift. In a two year study more than half were helped and of these forty per cent showed a fifty per cent improvement. It is thought that the stimulation modulates norepiphrine.' "

Depression had not been a major component in our experience of ME but it can be for some sufferers.

"This one is about bacteria in the gut." Lois nodded as she wrote. All three of our ME offspring changed their diet in order to help themselves get better. "One bacteria that was increased in number was the Roseburia."

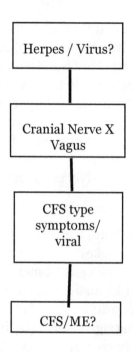

Herpes / Virus?

Cranial Nerve X
Vagus

CFS type
symptoms/
viral

CFS/ME?

Van Elkazzer Hypothesis.
A viral infection of the Vagus Nerve could cause Chronic
Fatigue Syndrome/ Myalgic Encephalomyelitis.

"What does that do?"

"Contributes to the production of energy and protects against gut inflammation."

I had made a batch of brownies, and as Jane was deep in her copy of *Breakthrough* and Lois was writing, I chose suitable mugs. 'Keep calm and carry on' for Jane, and a Rennie Mackintosh for our thoroughly Scottish Lois. I placed the plate of chocolate slices in the middle of all the papers.

"You won't believe this!" Jane folded back her journal and turned it to face us.

She waited until I had joined them with our mugs of tea and she had an attentive audience.

"Massachusetts. *Vagus Nerve Infection?*" She paused dramatically.

Dr Van Elzakker from Tufts University postulates that a viral or bacterial infection causes activation of glial cells, which support and protect nerve cells, somewhere along the Vagus nerve." Jane skipped to further down the article. "Glial cell activation produces inflammatory substances which bombard the Vagus nerve sending signals to the brain triggering myalgia, fever, sleep architecture changes and cognitive abnormalities.

She looked up to enjoy our expressions. The answer had been under our finger tips for over a year. The report was from autumn 2013, and, of course, I would have read it. Like all information that is not readily useful, it had just been filed away, literally and cranially.

"¡Es increíble!" said Lois who resorted to Spanish in moments of high crisis.

Were all the parts of the jigsaw falling into place?

"Van Elzakker says that depending on where the Vagus was affected would explain the various symptoms." She looked up at us both.

"How can we find out more?" Lois asked. She was understandably now more interested in CFS/ME than her labyrinthitis since she had recovered from the latter but her daughter still had ME.

"Use my computer." I advised Lois. She started a search while Jane read out the final part of the article.

"One advantage of the theory is that it simplifies the quest to find specific infectious causes for CFS/ME." Jane put down the journal.

"Any luck with the search, Lois?"

"No."

25 PACE Trial

Until this moment I had maintained, or tried to maintain, a professional and clinical approach to the Vagus story. Suddenly the force of its implications set off a reaction for which I had only one solution. Once I was alone, and able to, I donned my boots, coat, hat and gloves, and set off up the hill.

Behind our house the climb to a trig point is through four gates. It takes about twenty minutes of laboured breathing, unless it is a good day.

Even if we could not find Van Elzakker it was almost good enough to know that someone had come up with a comprehensive theory for ME. It was not that other great doctors had not done so already, E. D. Acheson, Melvin Ramsay, Byron Hyde, John Richardson to name a few had compiled their observations and produced evidence that ME was a biological illness. However they were either ahead of their time and the necessary technical progress had not been made, or their work had been adversely affected by the prominence in high places of psychiatrists who attributed ME to a state of mind following a viral infection and who changed the name to CFS. The label then encompassed any unexplained condition where fatigue was a factor. This lobby has been so powerful that for thirty years there have been only limited investigations into biological causation of ME.

By concentrating on fatigue in CFS many people have been misdiagnosed and their true illness neglected. By concentrating on fatigue all the other, often more debilitating, symptoms, have been ignored, and finally by concentrating on fatigue, the illness has been trivialised. By concentrating on dizziness and vertigo in labyrinthitis diagnosticians have not given equal weight to the other symptoms.

When comparing labyrinthitis and CFS both appear to be umbrella terms under whose label a collection of inexplicable but similar conditions had been dumped. The first have dizziness in common and the second, fatigue.

The treatment strategies for labyrinthitis and CFS also have parallels. Both have been considered to have a psychological overlay by some sections of the medical profession for which they have been prescribed CBT. In both conditions some medical professionals have stated that there is no basis for the patients to believe that they are suffering from a physical disease. Finally, both have had promoted as treatment the very movements or activities that these patients had gone to their doctors complaining that they were unable to do. In neither case were the results impressive, and if they were successful they were only so after *months* of 'treatment', when it is possible that the patient might have been at that stage of recovery without treatment.

The consequence of ignoring the other symptoms and treating the patient by prescribing exercise, made the patient *feel* worse in the cases of labyrinthitis, or *become* worse, in cases of CSF. Many labyrinth patients might have been spared unnecessary spells of vertigo, if they had not been compliant with the Cawthorne-Cooksey exercise regime. Many CFS/ME patients might have been saved unnecessary suffering if they had not been compliant with exercise regimes. It might be possible now to prove that patients had every reason to hold their beliefs that there was something seriously physically wrong with them.

As I trudged up the hill, barely noticing the sheep who lazily took themselves out of my path, a litany revolved around my head; Sophia Mirza, Emily Collingridge, Lynn Gilderdale; the names of three thirty-year-olds who had died of ME. The first two from the consequences of severe ME and the third by assisted suicide when she could suffer no longer. All died a lengthy agonising death that might have been prevented with better understanding and a great deal more compassion.

Yet do not blame the doctors. Doctors who think independently and prescribe rest and 'TLC' can see their careers ruined. These are extreme cases of ME. However, children and adults are regularly advised, cajoled or are unwittingly compliant with exercise regimes which make them worse.

Many patients, knowing this, are fearful of exercise. Survey after survey of ME patients has shown the deleterious effect of exercise, yet a trial, called the PACE* trial, conducted by psychiatrists between 2005 and 2011, persuaded the General

Medical Council that exercise was helpful in managing CFS/ ME. As recently as 2015, another analysis of the data gathered by the PACE trial concluded that fear avoidance beliefs were a major factor in the success or failure of exercise as treatment. They decided that if cognitive behaviour therapy was directed towards addressing this fear, the person would recover.

I reached the trig point and rested my elbows on the concrete pillar. I could hardly contain the sense of urgency I felt for ME patients to have this issue resolved and for them to have the right to rest and recover endorsed by the medical establishment. I wanted them to have the right to take months, if necessary, as our children had done, to get better.

It seemed beyond belief that the medical profession, who had had reports of this disease since the 1930s including observations and treatment possibilities from the findings of many diligent researchers, still followed a group of psychiatrists.

It seemed shocking enough that labyrinth patients were undergoing exercises and manoeuvres for crystals in their otoliths when there is no record of anyone ever having seen these crystals. It was even more extraordinary that people who go to a doctor complaining that they cannot exercise, should be assumed that they want to avoid exercise.

As more and more of the general public see for themselves that ME patients are not shirking, as newspapers report on celebrities who have succumbed to CFS/ME and then recovered, and as numerous pockets of research gain momentum, the established view of ME must change.

I climbed the gate, too idle to open the stiff unyielding metal catches, and cruised easily down the homeward stretch of farm road. I hoped fervently that the Massachusetts' theory, combining as it did all that is known about CFS/ME, might be the catalyst. If it was, then it would attract enough attention and research to spur on and fund new projects to find an answer to CFS/ME, and in the process find a new approach to labyrinthitis.

*PACE trial of four management strategies for CFS.
P=standard specialised medical care; A=adaptive pacing therapy;
C=cognitive behavioural therapy; G=graded exercise therapy

Jane left a message on my phone. "I've found him!"

"I googled *Doctor* Van Elzakker," Jane began, excited, not allowing me to interrupt. "Doctor Michael Van Elzakker is a neuro-scientist in Massachusetts. He was desperate to tell everybody about his theory of an infection of the Vagus nerve and went on until someone would listen! He understands ME because he has a friend with CFS/ME and knows it is not psychological." Her words were tumbling out.

"*'Does the Vagus give a possible reason for all the symptoms and signs of CFS/ME.'* That's the crux of the matter, isn't it? It has to cover everything." Jane said that she had the information from an interview that Dr Van Elzakker had given.

"The Vagus is the reason that we get ill during any illness. It is its job to heal and repair and being ill is how we get better, if that makes sense. The Vagus is a mixed cranial nerve, both motor and sensory. Its parasympathetic influence over the body results from motor activity; its function in detecting peripheral infection and triggering sickness behaviour results from sensory activity. It isn't as if the parasympathetic is overactive and the sympathetic underactive, they switch on and off responding to information and sending out signals as necessary. What matters is whether the Vagus can respond to signals appropriately."

Jane went on.

"He needs PET scans of the Vagus nerve to prove his theory but they cost thousands of pounds. PET scans are done regularly on the brain but they would need to go a bit lower, to the medulla, and they would need to do a lot of them."

Jane then said that the interviewer asked about targeting antibodies with radio-labelling so as to find clusters of infection. "Van Elzakker said that it was not possible because they don't know which antibodies are responsible and if you do choose one, say HHV6 or EBV4 then may be the patient has the other one, or has them in their system anyway. Besides, he said, the Vagus is huge, and they could be anywhere, and because antibodies cannot always get into the ganglia, they might not find the source anyway."

"The interviewer asked why anti-virals might not work when herpes love sensory ganglia and it would seem logical that that is where they could be targeted. Van Elzakker replied that the Central Nervous System has a blood brain barrier which makes it difficult for the immune system to infiltrate, and this is the same for the rest of the nervous system, it is 'immunoprivileged'. That means it makes it difficult for our own immune system to fight infection there. It is equally difficult for drugs to try and fight infection there."

I interrupted her. "Cytokines are something in the blood that doctors monitor to see if there is an infection in the body. Dr Mady Hornig has reported finding cytokines in the blood of ME patients, provided that they have been ill for less than three years, which she says proves that there is an infection."

"Yes. Cytokines are immune molecules which are important in cell signalling. They are released by cells and affect the behaviour of immune responses. However they rarely find cytokines in ME patients and Van Elzakker explained that cytokines are difficult to find because the laboratory techniques are complicated. He said that just because the tests come back negative it does not mean that there is no infection."

"There was some scepticism by the psychiatrists about the cytokine findings." I observed.

"Other trials will have to be undertaken. Also, for example, in lung infections increased cytokine levels in the blood will probably not be found because it is a local infection. The Vagus infection would be a local infection. Cytokines may only be found if the infection is very severe."

Jane kept her best bit of news until last; it was not about research but about CFS/ME itself and concerned the very crux of the CFS/ME controversy regarding graded exercise and cognitive behavioural therapy.

"Van Elzakker commented on how CBT helps some ME patients. He said that about 30% receive some benefit. Stress causes a cytokine response, and patients fear exercise because they know that it will make them worse. This fear is justified, it does make them worse, but if it makes them unable to function at all, then CBT can benefit people who need to know what is a sensible level. So three out of ten are helped."

"He said that they are justified in thinking that exercise makes them worse?" I repeated.

"He says that the PACE trial is 'infamous' because it assumed that fear avoidance was the *cause* of ME." She slowed down.

> Exercise causes muscle tissue to produce pro-inflammatory cytokine IL6. This would exacerbate a local cytokine response in Vagus Nerve ganglia or in any ganglia nearby. If there is already an ongoing infection, exercise would make them worse.

Neither of us spoke for quite a while. This finding, if accepted by the medical profession, would change the lives of ME patients. Here was a physiological reason for avoiding exercise.

Jane read out the last part of the interview.

> Those of us who think that CFS is not psychological tend to think there's an immune dysfunction of some sort. Looking for cytokines is an obvious potential link between the immune system and CFS.

"Van Elzakker also said that if the theory is correct, then it could explain the mystery about how a virus might trigger an illness and then seem to disappear."

It was a lot to take in.

Finally I said. "And all because of your Vagus nerve, Jane!"

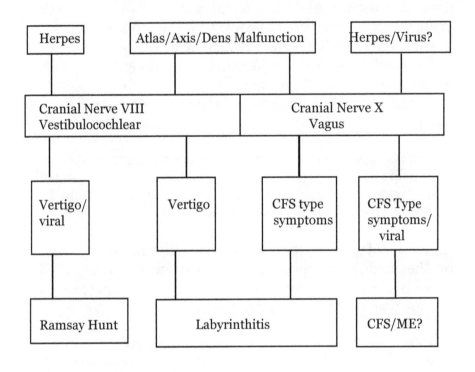

Herpes	Atlas/Axis/Dens Malfunction	Herpes/Virus?

Cranial Nerve VIII Vestibulocochlear	Cranial Nerve X Vagus

Vertigo/ viral	Vertigo	CFS type symptoms	CFS Type symptoms/ viral

Ramsay Hunt	Labyrinthitis	CFS/ME?

Viral infection or mechanical malfunction causing pressure in the area of the atlas/axis/medulla results in symptoms of Ramsay Hunt Syndrome or Labyrinthitis or Chronic Fatigue Syndrome / Myalgic Encephalomyelitis

27   Epilogue

The possibility that a virus of the Vagus could cause ME/CFS has the potential to confirm that those symptoms of labyrinthitis which resemble ME/CFS can be caused by mechanical pressure on the Vagus nerve.

It is not that the Vagus itself causes dizziness and vertigo, but the Vagus could cause the ME/CFS-like symptoms that are experienced by labyrinthitis patients along with their vertigo.

Whether the cause is infection or musculo-skeletal pressure, the fact that the vestibulocochlear and the Vagus can be affected by both mechanisms is reason to believe that labyrinthitis and ME/CFS can be attributed to dysfunctions of cranial nerves that are in the same anatomical area.

To fully solve the conundrum of Lois's vertigo including all the other symptoms of labyrinthitis the outcome of the Massachusetts investigations is necessary. Only then will all four of the components that could cause ME/CFS and labyrinthitis be present.

It seemed like an anti-climax. We had explored the story of labyrinthitis, but all three of us were, if we were honest, much more concerned about CFS/ME. Instead of a triumphant 'eureka', it felt like the edge of a cliff. A long pause, indefinitely long, before the plunge into the sea of science. If only the rivers of science were not so long. If only they could all flow into one ocean. If only all the necessary experts could be enticed to come together to solve the problem of ME.

ME must be one of the most intriguing challenges that faces medicine if only because of the numbers of people affected. A quarter of a million in the UK alone. When the many months, and years, of suffering are taken into account, ME must be rated as one of the most devastating illnesses.

In the last century most childhood illnesses have been eradicated or at least minimised. Malaria is now contained, AIDS victims are no longer, in the western world, under an immediate sentence of death, and cancer victims are having better than ever expectations of a cure or prolonged lives.

Diseases affecting fewer patients, such as Cystic Fibrosis, Type 1 Diabetes, Multiple Sclerosis and Parkinson's, have had extensively researched diagnostic and treatment regimes, whereas CFS/ME has been sidelined.

If it had not been for papers by a psychiatrist in the 1970s which encouraged scepticism and disrupted the momentum of interest in ME, scientific studies begun in 1934 might well have yielded good results by now. When the medical profession is baffled by inexplicable symptoms which endure and persist, they tend to fall back on psychosomatic explanations. Parkinson's was once dismissed as a suppression of excess libido, and Multiple Sclerosis as hysteria, until proved otherwise by research. The psychological explanation for CFS/ME is hopefully on the brink of being refuted.

A young girl called Devina became ill in 1999 aged thirteen. Two years later she was well on the road to recovery thanks to intuitively good nursing by her mother, and a sympathetic and accommodating school. At this point her consultant prescribed graded exercise therapy. Her physiotherapist interpreted this as rehabilitation in the gym, increasing her level of activity. Davina, keen to comply, exercised.

She became ill again, worse than she had been in the previous two years. She never recovered. She is now housebound spending her days recumbent. She has pain, malaise and nausea. Her cognitive ability is so impaired that she cannot read for more than five or ten minutes. She can watch television in small amounts.

Davina writes, by speaking into her phone, for three or four minutes on the days that she is well enough. She is now thirty. She has watched her sisters complete university, find rewarding jobs, and marry. She maintains the hope that one day she will be well.

"Do you think ME is contagious?" Jane asked in a recent conversation.

"There are no facts to support this possibility because ME is not a recognised illness and statistics are not available, but the Royal Free epidemic indicates that it can be. Doctors do not want to investigate an illness that is purported to be psychological and which, if they acted otherwise, might reflect on their career. Two doctors have had their careers threatened because they had prescribed rest, or gave prescriptions, for CFS/ME."

"Can anyone get ME?" Jane persisted.

"It's the only way to think. If it is a virus, we are all susceptible. If it is herpes, then we are all harbouring it, and it could be activated at any time."

"So no-one is safe?"

"Given the wrong circumstances, anyone could get ME. Given poor advice, financial constraints, unlucky family circumstances, anyone with ME could go on to develop severe ME. Patients describe this as a living death. None of us has immunity from ME. We are all vulnerable."

"But Van Elzakker's theory puts forward another avenue of exploration into the cause of ME."

"And hopefully a cure!"

Jane responded with her favourite mantra.

"Never Ever Give Up!"

References

Books:

Green, J.H. *Basic Clinical Physiology*, 3ed, Oxford Medical
  Publications, 2002
Ford, Gail, and Marsden, Jon, *Handbook of Vestibular
  Re- education* (based on Cawthorne & Cooksey 1945),
  University College of London, 2006
Ginsberg, Lionel, *Lecture Notes in Neurology*, 9ed Wiley-
  Blackwell, 2010
Hyde, Byron, *Missed Diagnoses in Myalgic
  Encephalomyelitis and Chronic Fatigue Syndrome*,
  Nightingale Foundation, 2ed, Lulu 2011
Luxon, Linda, *Theoretical basis of physical exercise regimes
  and manoeuvres*, in Luxon and Davies, eds, *Handbook of
  Vestibular Rehabilitation*, Wiley, 2006
Ramsay, A Melvin, *Myalgic Encephalomyelitis and Post Viral
  Fatigue States: The Saga of the Royal Free Disease*, 2ed,
  Gower Medical, 1988
Sapolsky, Robert M., *Why Zebras Don't Get Ulcers* 3ed, W H
  Freeman and Company, 1998
Williams and Warwick, *Gray's Anatomy*, 36ed, Churchill
  Livingstone, 1980

Journals:

Breakthrough Journal of ME Research UK Issues 18-21
Hunt, Richard, *Herpes Viruses,* Virology Chapter 11,
  University of South Carolina, 2016.
  http://www.microbiologybook.org/virol/herpes.htm
Richardson, John, *Viral Isolation from Brain in Myalgic
  Encephalomyelitis* Journal of CFS 2001: 9 (3-4) 15-19
Twisk FN, Maes M. *A review on cognitive behavorial therapy
  (CBT) and graded exercise therapy (GET) in myalgic
  encephalomyelitis (ME) / chronic fatigue syndrome (CFS):
  CBT/GET is not only ineffective and not evidence-based,*

but also potentially harmful for many patients with ME/CFS. Neuro Endocrinol Lett (August 2009) 30 (3): 284–299.

Van Elzakker, Michael *Chronic Fatigue Syndrome from Vagus Nerve Infection: a psychoneuroimmunological hypothesis* Medical Hypotheses 81 (2013) 414-423 PubMed Elsevier

Walker, Andrew, P*hysiotherapist's practice in the management of anxiety in patients with vestibular disorders,* Frontline Physiotherapy Journal 18 Nov 2015

White PD, Sharpe MC, Chalder T, DeCesare JC, Walwyn R. *Protocol for the PACE trial: A randomised controlled trial of adaptive pacing, cognitive behaviour therapy, and graded exercise as supplements to standardised specialist medical care versus standardised specialist medical care alone for patients with the chronic fatigue syndrome/myalgic encephalomyelitis or encephalopathy.* BMC Neurol, 2007 7:6